THE HEALTHY GUT DIET BOOK FOR WOMEN

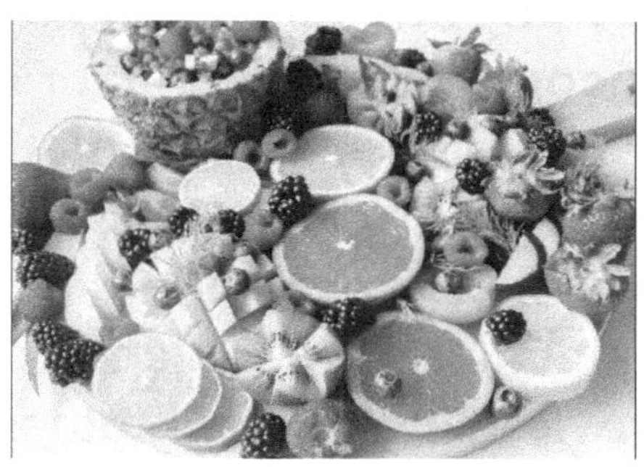

"A Guide to Nourishing Your Gut for Vibrant Health"

EMMA LYNCH

TABLE OF CONTENTS

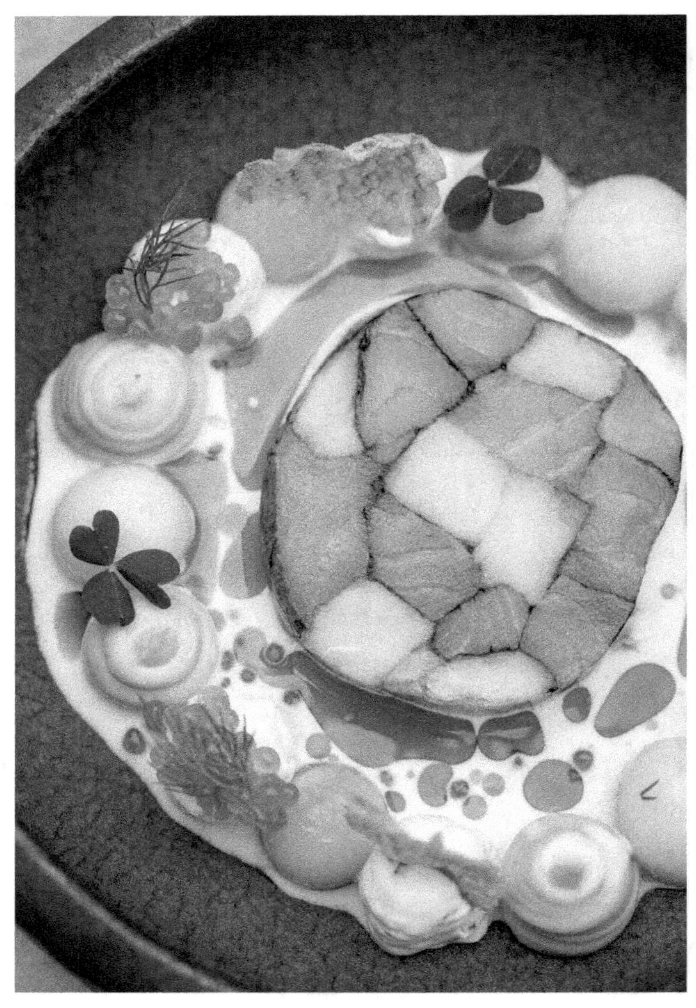

INTRODUCTION

Welcome to "The Healthy Gut Diet Book For Women:" In this comprehensive book, we embark on a journey to explore the intricate relationship between gut health and overall well-being, with a focus tailored specifically for the unique needs of women. As we delve into the fascinating world of digestive wellness, we aim to empower women to take control of their health and vitality through nourishing their gut.

WHY A HEALTHY GUT MATTERS FOR WOMEN

A healthy gut is essential for women due to its profound impact on various aspects of their overall health and well-being. Here are several reasons why gut health matters specifically for women:

1. Hormonal Balance: The gut microbiome plays a crucial role in metabolizing and regulating hormones, including estrogen and progesterone. Imbalances in these hormones can lead to issues such as irregular menstruation, PMS, and fertility problems. By maintaining a healthy gut, women can support optimal hormonal balance, promoting reproductive health and overall well-being.

2. Digestive Health: Women are more prone to certain digestive disorders such as irritable bowel syndrome (IBS) and inflammatory bowel disease (IBD). A healthy gut helps to maintain proper digestion, absorption of nutrients, and regular bowel movements, reducing the risk of gastrointestinal issues and promoting gut comfort.

3. Immune Function: Approximately 70% of the body's immune cells are located in the gut-associated lymphoid tissue (GALT). A healthy gut microbiome supports a robust immune system, helping to defend against infections, autoimmune diseases, and other immune-related conditions that disproportionately affect women.

4. Mental Health: The gut-brain axis, a bidirectional communication network between the gut and the brain, plays a significant role in regulating mood and mental health. Women are more likely to experience conditions such as anxiety and depression, which have been linked to imbalances in gut bacteria and inflammation in the gut. By nurturing a healthy gut, women can support their mental well-being and emotional resilience.

5. Weight Management: Hormonal fluctuations, especially during menstruation, pregnancy, and menopause, can influence appetite, metabolism, and body composition. A balanced gut microbiome helps regulate energy metabolism and appetite, making it easier for women to maintain a healthy weight and prevent obesity-related health issues.

6. Skin Health: Conditions such as acne, eczema, and psoriasis are influenced by both hormonal imbalances and inflammation in the body. A healthy gut microbiome helps to regulate inflammation and support skin health, promoting a clear, radiant complexion.

Overall, prioritizing gut health is essential for women to support their hormonal balance, digestive health, immune function, mental well-being, weight management, and skin health. By adopting a healthy gut diet and lifestyle habits that nurture the gut microbiome, women can optimize their health and thrive in all aspects of life.

OVERVIEW OF THE BOOK

In this comprehensive guide, "The Healthy Gut Diet Book For Women," we embark on a journey to explore the intricate connection between gut health and women's well-being. Through this book, we aim to provide a holistic approach to digestive wellness tailored specifically for women, offering practical advice, delicious recipes, and evidence-based strategies to support optimal gut health.

The book is divided into several sections, each addressing key aspects of gut health and its significance for women's health:

1. Understanding Gut Health: We begin by laying the foundation with an exploration of what gut health entails, including the role of the gut microbiome, factors influencing gut health, and the importance of maintaining a balanced ecosystem within the digestive tract.

2. The Basics of a Healthy Gut Diet: Next, we delve into the fundamentals of a healthy gut diet, highlighting key nutrients, foods to include, and those to avoid for optimal digestive wellness. We emphasize the importance of fiber, probiotics, and prebiotics, as well as provide practical tips for meal planning and preparation.

3. Creating a Gut-Healthy Meal Plan: This section offers guidance on crafting personalized meal plans tailored to individual preferences and lifestyles. We provide sample meal plans and offer suggestions for incorporating gut-healthy foods into daily menus, making it easier for women to nourish their bodies and support digestive health.

4. Gut-Healthy Recipes for Women: With a collection of mouthwatering recipes, we demonstrate how delicious and satisfying a gut-healthy diet can be. From nourishing breakfasts to flavorful lunches, dinners, snacks, and beverages, these recipes are designed to appeal to women's tastes while promoting digestive wellness.

5. Lifestyle Factors for Gut Health: Recognizing the interconnectedness of mind, body, and gut, we explore the role of lifestyle factors such as stress management, sleep, and exercise in supporting gut health. We offer practical strategies for integrating these lifestyle habits into daily routines to promote overall well-being.

6. Special Considerations for Women's Health: This section addresses specific considerations for women's health, including the impact of hormonal fluctuations on gut health, pregnancy, and menopause. We provide guidance on how women can support their digestive wellness during various stages of life.

7. Supplements for Gut Health: Finally, we discuss the role of supplements in complementing a healthy gut diet and offer recommendations for selecting and incorporating supplements to address specific digestive concerns and optimize gut health.

Throughout the book, readers will find evidence-based information, practical tips, and actionable steps to empower them to take control of their digestive wellness and thrive from the inside out. Whether you're looking to address digestive issues, support hormonal balance, or simply optimize your overall health, "The Healthy Gut Diet Book For Women" provides the guidance and inspiration you need to nourish your gut and transform your health journey.

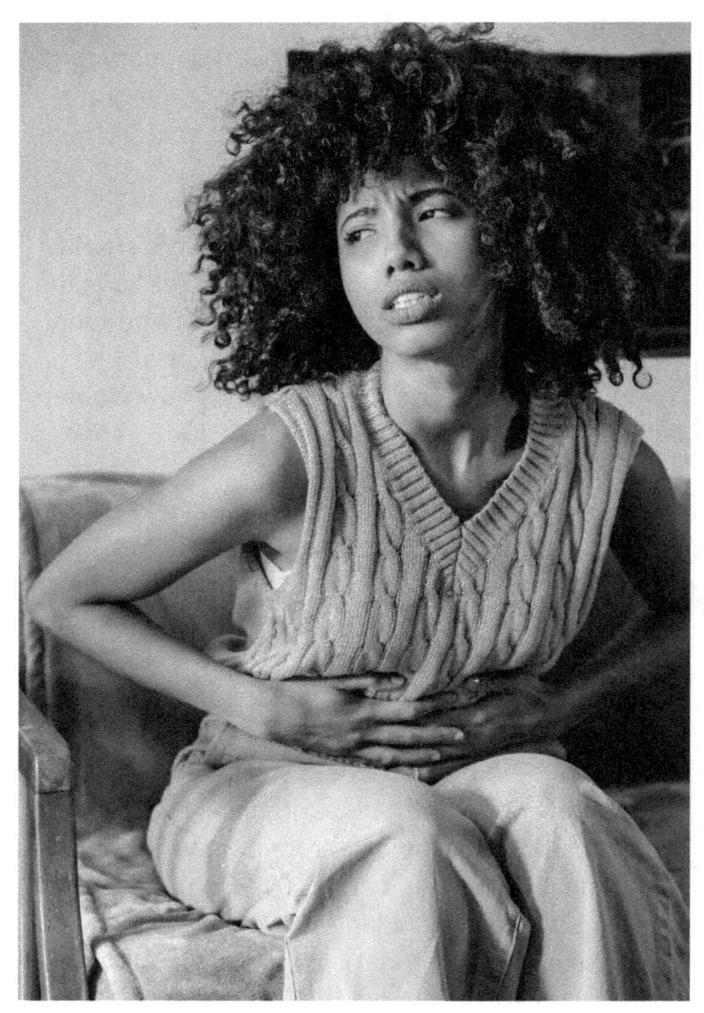

CHAPTER ONE

UNDERSTANDING GUT HEALTH

Gut health has become increasingly popular in recent years, and for good reason. The gut, often referred to as the body's "second brain," plays a vital role in overall health and well-being. In this section, we will delve into what gut health is, the importance of the gut microbiome, factors influencing gut health, and the significance of maintaining a balanced ecosystem within the digestive tract.

1. What is Gut Health?

Gut health encompasses the function and balance of the gastrointestinal tract, including the stomach, small intestine, and large intestine. It involves the efficient digestion and absorption of nutrients, the maintenance of a healthy gut lining, and the regulation of immune function within the gut.

2. The Gut Microbiome

At the heart of gut health lies the gut microbiome, a complex ecosystem of trillions of microorganisms, including bacteria, viruses, fungi, and archaea, that inhabit the digestive tract. These microbes play a crucial role in various physiological processes, such as digestion, metabolism, immune function, and even mood regulation.

3. Factors Influencing Gut Health

Several factors can influence the balance and diversity of the gut microbiome, including diet, lifestyle, medications, stress, and environmental exposures. Poor dietary choices, such as diets high in processed foods and low in fiber, can disrupt the delicate balance of gut bacteria, leading to dysbiosis and increased susceptibility to digestive disorders and chronic diseases.

4. Maintaining a Balanced Gut Ecosystem

A balanced gut ecosystem is characterized by a diverse array of beneficial bacteria that work in harmony to support digestive health and overall well-being. Key components of maintaining a healthy gut ecosystem include consuming a diet rich in fiber, fermented foods, and prebiotics; minimizing exposure to antibiotics and other medications that can disrupt gut flora; managing stress levels; and avoiding environmental toxins.

By understanding the fundamentals of gut health, women can take proactive steps to support their digestive wellness and optimize their overall health and vitality. In the following sections, we will explore practical strategies for implementing a healthy gut diet, creating gut-healthy meal plans, and addressing specific considerations for women's health. Through education and empowerment, we can harness the power of gut health to nourish our bodies from within and thrive in all aspects of life.

THE GUT MICROBIOME

The gut microbiome is a complex and diverse ecosystem of microorganisms that reside in the gastrointestinal tract, primarily in the large intestine. Comprising trillions of bacteria, viruses, fungi, and other microbes, the gut microbiome plays a crucial role in maintaining overall health and well-being. In this section, we will explore the significance of the gut microbiome, its composition, functions, and factors that influence its balance.

1. Composition of the Gut Microbiome:

The gut microbiome is composed of thousands of different species of bacteria, each with its own unique characteristics and functions. The predominant phyla of bacteria in the gut include Firmicutes, Bacteroidetes, Actinobacteria, and Proteobacteria. These bacteria work synergistically to perform essential functions such as fermenting dietary fiber, producing vitamins and short-chain fatty acids, and regulating immune function.

2. Functions of the Gut Microbiome:

The gut microbiome plays a multitude of roles in maintaining health and homeostasis within the body. Some key functions of the gut microbiome include:

- Digestion and metabolism: Gut bacteria assist in the breakdown and fermentation of dietary fibers and complex carbohydrates, producing nutrients and short-chain fatty acids that nourish the cells lining the intestine.

- **Immune regulation:** The gut microbiome interacts with the immune system, helping to train and modulate immune responses and protect against pathogens.

- **Synthesis of vitamins and other bioactive compounds:** Certain gut bacteria produce vitamins such as vitamin K and biotin, as well as neurotransmitters and other metabolites that influence various physiological processes.

- **Maintenance of gut barrier function:** Gut bacteria contribute to the integrity of the gut barrier, preventing the translocation of harmful substances from the gut into the bloodstream.

3. Factors Influencing the Gut Microbiome:

The composition and diversity of the gut microbiome can be influenced by various factors, including diet, lifestyle, medications, environmental exposures, and genetics. Dietary factors such as fiber intake, consumption of fermented foods, and the balance of macronutrients can significantly impact the composition of gut bacteria. Additionally, factors such as stress, antibiotics, and exposure to environmental toxins can disrupt the delicate balance of the gut microbiome, leading to dysbiosis and associated health issues.

Understanding the importance of the gut microbiome and its role in maintaining health is essential for women's well-being. In the following sections, we will explore strategies for nurturing a healthy gut microbiome through diet, lifestyle modifications, and targeted interventions. By supporting the diversity and balance of gut bacteria, women can optimize their digestive health, immune function, and overall vitality.

FACTORS AFFECTING GUT HEALTH IN WOMEN

Gut health is influenced by a myriad of factors, and women may experience unique challenges and considerations that impact the balance and function of their gut microbiome. In this section, we will explore some of the key factors affecting gut health in women and how they can optimize their digestive wellness.

1. Hormonal Fluctuations:

Hormonal changes throughout a woman's life, including puberty, menstruation, pregnancy, and menopause, can have a significant impact on gut health. Estrogen and progesterone, in particular, play a role in regulating gut motility, immune function, and the composition of gut bacteria. Fluctuations in hormone levels can contribute to digestive issues such as bloating, constipation, or diarrhea. Women may benefit from adopting strategies to support hormonal balance, such as maintaining a healthy weight, managing stress, and optimizing nutrition.

2. Menstrual Cycle:

The menstrual cycle can influence gut function and symptoms of digestive discomfort in some women. Changes in hormone levels during different phases of the menstrual cycle may affect gut motility, water retention, and sensitivity to certain foods. Some women may experience digestive symptoms such as bloating or abdominal discomfort during the premenstrual phase. Strategies such as maintaining a balanced diet, staying hydrated, and managing stress can help alleviate menstrual-related digestive issues.

3. Oral Contraceptives and Hormone Replacement Therapy:

The use of oral contraceptives and hormone replacement therapy (HRT) can impact gut health by altering hormone levels and potentially affecting the composition of gut bacteria. Some women may experience digestive side effects such as nausea, bloating, or changes in bowel habits when starting or discontinuing hormonal medications. It's essential for women to discuss any concerns or symptoms with their healthcare provider and explore strategies to support gut health while using hormonal medications.

4. Pregnancy:

Pregnancy is a unique physiological state that can profoundly influence gut health. Hormonal changes, increased progesterone levels, and changes in dietary habits during pregnancy can affect digestion and bowel function. Additionally, pregnancy-related conditions such as gestational diabetes and preeclampsia can impact gut health and increase the risk of certain digestive issues. Pregnant women can benefit from consuming a balanced diet rich in fiber, staying hydrated, and incorporating probiotic-rich foods to support digestive wellness during pregnancy.

5. Menopause:
The hormonal changes associated with menopause can impact gut health and increase the risk of digestive issues such as constipation, bloating, and irritable bowel syndrome (IBS). Declining estrogen levels may alter gut motility and increase inflammation in the gut, contributing to digestive discomfort. Women transitioning through menopause can benefit from adopting a gut-healthy diet, managing stress, and incorporating lifestyle strategies to support hormonal balance and digestive wellness.

By understanding the unique factors affecting gut health in women, individuals can take proactive steps to optimize their digestive wellness and overall well-being. Through a combination of dietary modifications, lifestyle interventions, and targeted support, women can nurture a healthy gut microbiome and enjoy vibrant health at every stage of life.

CHAPTER TWO

THE BASICS OF A HEALTHY GUT DIET

A healthy gut diet is essential for maintaining optimal gut health and overall well-being. In this section, we will explore the key components of a healthy gut diet, including the nutrients, foods to include, and those to avoid for supporting digestive wellness.

1. Fiber-Rich Foods:

Dietary fiber is essential for promoting gut health as it helps to regulate bowel movements, support the growth of beneficial gut bacteria, and reduce the risk of digestive issues such as constipation and diverticulosis. Women should aim to consume a variety of fiber-rich foods, including fruits, vegetables, whole grains, legumes, nuts, and seeds, to ensure an adequate intake of both soluble and insoluble fiber.

2. Probiotic Foods:

Probiotics are beneficial bacteria that can help to maintain a healthy balance of gut flora and support digestive function. Women can incorporate probiotic-rich foods such as yogurt, kefir, fermented vegetables (e.g., sauerkraut, kimchi), kombucha, and miso into their diet to promote the growth of beneficial gut bacteria and support immune function.

3. Prebiotic Foods:

Prebiotics are non-digestible fibers that serve as fuel for beneficial gut bacteria, helping to stimulate their growth and activity. Women can include prebiotic-rich foods such as garlic, onions, leeks, asparagus, bananas, oats, and Jerusalem artichokes in their diet to support the proliferation of beneficial gut bacteria and enhance digestive health.

4. Lean Proteins:

Protein is an essential nutrient for overall health and muscle repair, but the source and quality of protein can impact gut health. Women should focus on consuming lean sources of protein such as poultry, fish, tofu, legumes, and eggs, while limiting intake of red and processed meats, which may be detrimental to gut health and increase the risk of colorectal cancer.

5. Healthy Fats:

Healthy fats, such as those found in avocados, nuts, seeds, olive oil, and fatty fish, are important for supporting heart health, brain function, and hormone production. Including these sources of healthy fats in the diet can help to reduce inflammation in the gut and support the absorption of fat-soluble vitamins, such as vitamin D and vitamin E.

6. Hydration:

Adequate hydration is essential for maintaining proper digestion and bowel function. Women should aim to drink plenty of water throughout the day to prevent dehydration and support optimal digestive health. Herbal teas, coconut water, and infused water with fruits or herbs can also contribute to hydration while providing additional nutrients and antioxidants.

7. Foods to Limit or Avoid:

Certain foods and dietary habits can negatively impact gut health and contribute to digestive discomfort and inflammation. Women should limit or avoid highly processed foods, sugary snacks and beverages, artificial sweeteners, fried foods, excessive alcohol consumption, and foods high in saturated and trans fats.

By focusing on incorporating nutrient-dense, whole foods into their diet and avoiding processed and inflammatory foods, women can support digestive wellness and promote a healthy gut microbiome. In the following sections, we will explore practical tips for meal planning, creating gut-healthy recipes, and implementing lifestyle strategies to optimize gut health and overall well-being.

KEY COMPONENT OF A HEALTHY GUT DIET

The following are some key components of a healthy gut diet.

1. Fiber: Dietary fiber is essential for maintaining a healthy gut as it promotes regular bowel movements, supports the growth of beneficial gut bacteria, and helps prevent constipation and other digestive issues. Incorporate fiber-rich foods such as fruits, vegetables, whole grains, legumes, nuts, and seeds into your daily diet.

2. Probiotics: Probiotics are beneficial bacteria that help maintain a balanced gut microbiome and support digestive health. Include probiotic-rich foods like yogurt, kefir, fermented vegetables (such as sauerkraut and kimchi), kombucha, and miso in your diet.

3. Prebiotics: Prebiotics are non-digestible fibers that serve as food for beneficial gut bacteria, helping them thrive and multiply. Prebiotic-rich foods include Jerusalem artichokes, garlic, onions, leeks, asparagus, bananas, and oats.

4. Lean Proteins: Opt for lean sources of protein such as poultry, fish, tofu, legumes, and eggs. These protein sources are easier to digest and support muscle repair and growth without contributing to gut inflammation.

5. Healthy Fats: Include sources of healthy fats in your diet, such as avocados, nuts, seeds, olive oil, and fatty fish like salmon and mackerel. These fats are anti-inflammatory and support the absorption of fat-soluble vitamins, which are essential for overall health.

6. Hydration: Stay hydrated by drinking plenty of water throughout the day. Hydration is crucial for maintaining proper digestion, supporting bowel movements, and preventing constipation. Herbal teas, coconut water, and fruit or herb-infused water are all great ways to stay hydrated.

7. Whole Foods: Focus on consuming whole, minimally processed foods that are rich in nutrients and free from artificial additives and preservatives. These foods provide essential vitamins, minerals, and antioxidants that support gut health and overall well-being.

By incorporating these key components into your diet, you can nourish your gut, support a healthy gut microbiome, and promote optimal digestive function. Remember to prioritize variety, balance, and moderation in your food choices to achieve a well-rounded and sustainable healthy gut diet.

FOODS TO INCLUDE AND AVOID

The following are some food to include

1. Fiber-rich fruits and vegetables: Incorporate a variety of fruits and vegetables into your diet, such as berries, apples, oranges, broccoli, spinach, kale, and carrots. These foods are high in fiber, vitamins, minerals, and antioxidants, which support digestive health and overall well-being.

2. Whole grains: Choose whole grains such as oats, brown rice, quinoa, barley, and whole wheat bread and pasta. These grains are rich in fiber and nutrients that promote gut health and help regulate digestion.

3. Legumes: Include beans, lentils, chickpeas, and peas in your meals. Legumes are a great source of fiber, protein, and prebiotics, which nourish beneficial gut bacteria and support digestive function.

4. Fermented foods: Incorporate fermented foods into your diet, such as yogurt, kefir, sauerkraut, kimchi, kombucha, and miso. These foods are rich in probiotics, which help maintain a healthy balance of gut bacteria and support immune function.

5. Healthy fats: Include sources of healthy fats in your diet, such as avocados, nuts, seeds, olive oil, and fatty fish like salmon and mackerel. These fats are anti-inflammatory and support gut health and overall well-being.

6. Lean proteins: Choose lean sources of protein such as poultry, fish, tofu, tempeh, legumes, and eggs. These proteins are easier to digest and support muscle repair and growth without contributing to gut inflammation.

Foods to Avoid:

1. Highly processed foods: Limit your intake of processed foods such as sugary snacks, fast food, packaged snacks, and processed meats. These foods are often low in fiber and nutrients and may disrupt gut health and contribute to inflammation.

2. Sugary beverages: Reduce your consumption of sugary beverages such as soda, fruit juice, energy drinks, and sweetened coffee and tea. These beverages are high in sugar and may negatively impact gut health and increase the risk of chronic diseases.

3. Artificial sweeteners: Avoid artificial sweeteners such as aspartame, saccharin, sucralose, and acesulfame potassium. These sweeteners may alter gut bacteria composition and contribute to digestive issues and metabolic disorders.

4. Excessive alcohol: Limit your intake of alcohol, as excessive alcohol consumption can disrupt gut bacteria balance, increase intestinal permeability, and contribute to digestive issues such as inflammation and liver damage.

5. Fried and greasy foods: Minimize your consumption of fried and greasy foods, as they are often high in unhealthy fats and may contribute to digestive discomfort and inflammation.

6. Excessive salt: Reduce your intake of foods high in salt, such as processed meats, canned soups, and salty snacks. High salt intake can disrupt gut bacteria balance and increase the risk of digestive issues and cardiovascular disease.

By focusing on including nutrient-rich whole foods and avoiding processed and inflammatory foods, you can support a healthy gut microbiome, promote optimal digestive function, and enhance overall well-being. Remember to prioritize balance, variety, and moderation in your diet for long-term gut health and vitality.

IMPORTANCE OF FIBER, PROBIOTICS AND PREBIOTICS

The importance of fiber, probiotics, and prebiotics cannot be overstated when it comes to maintaining a healthy gut and overall well-being. Let's look at each of these components independently.

1. Fiber:
   - **Digestive health:** Fiber plays a crucial role in promoting regular bowel movements and preventing constipation by adding bulk to stool and facilitating its passage through the digestive tract.
   - **Gut microbiome:** Certain types of fiber, known as prebiotic fibers, serve as food for beneficial gut bacteria. By nourishing these bacteria, fiber helps to maintain a diverse and balanced gut microbiome, which is essential for digestive health and immune function.
   - **Heart health:** Soluble fiber found in foods like oats, beans, and fruits can help lower cholesterol levels and reduce the risk of heart disease by binding to cholesterol in the digestive tract and promoting its excretion.
   - **Blood sugar control:** Fiber slows down the absorption of sugar from the bloodstream, helping to stabilize blood sugar levels and reduce the risk of type 2 diabetes.

2. Probiotics:
   - **Gut health:** Probiotics are beneficial bacteria that colonize the gut and help maintain a healthy balance of microorganisms. They support digestion, nutrient absorption, and immune function, while also helping to prevent the growth of harmful bacteria.

- **Immune function:** Probiotics play a critical role in regulating immune responses in the gut and throughout the body. They help strengthen the intestinal barrier, stimulate the production of immune cells, and modulate inflammation, thereby supporting overall immune function.

- **Digestive disorders:** Probiotics have been shown to be beneficial in managing certain digestive disorders such as irritable bowel syndrome (IBS), inflammatory bowel disease (IBD), and antibiotic-associated diarrhea by restoring microbial balance and reducing symptoms.

3. Prebiotics:

- **Gut microbiome:** Prebiotics are non-digestible fibers that serve as food for beneficial gut bacteria. By nourishing these bacteria, prebiotics help promote the growth and activity of beneficial microbes, which in turn support digestive health, immune function, and overall well-being.

- **Digestive health:** Prebiotics help stimulate the production of short-chain fatty acids (SCFAs) in the gut, which provide energy to colon cells, improve intestinal barrier function, and reduce inflammation. This can help alleviate symptoms of digestive disorders such as constipation, diarrhea, and inflammatory bowel disease (IBD).

- **Weight management:** Some studies suggest that prebiotics may help regulate appetite, reduce calorie absorption, and promote the growth of beneficial gut bacteria associated with a healthy weight. This may have implications for weight management and metabolic health.

In summary, fiber, probiotics, and prebiotics are essential components of a healthy gut diet that support digestive health, immune function, and overall well-being. By incorporating these nutrients into your diet through a variety of whole foods and supplements, you can nurture a thriving gut microbiome and optimize your health from the inside out.

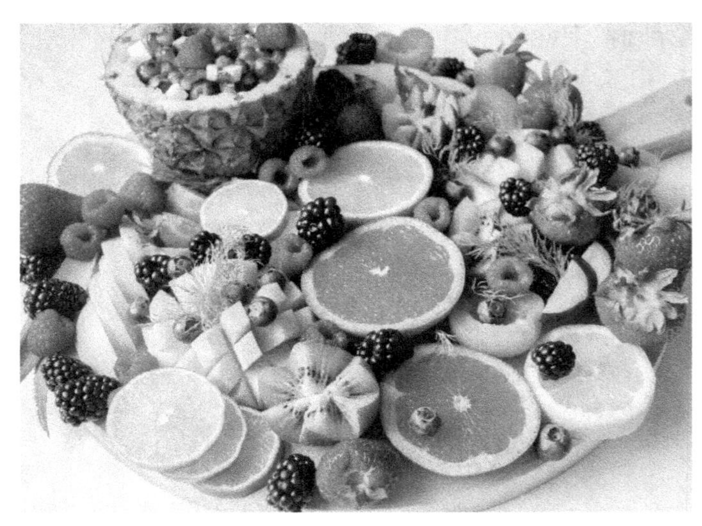

CHAPTER THREE

CREATING A GUT-HEALTHY MEAL PLAN

Creating a gut-healthy meal plan is an essential step in supporting digestive wellness and promoting overall health. Here are some guidelines and tips for crafting a gut-friendly meal plan:

1. Incorporate Fiber-Rich Foods:

- Include plenty of fruits, vegetables, whole grains, legumes, nuts, and seeds in your meals and snacks. These foods are rich in dietary fiber, which helps promote regular bowel movements, supports the growth of beneficial gut bacteria, and aids in digestion.

2. Include Probiotic-Rich Foods:

- Incorporate probiotic-rich foods such as yogurt, kefir, fermented vegetables (like sauerkraut and kimchi), kombucha, and miso into your diet. These foods contain beneficial bacteria that help maintain a healthy balance of gut flora and support digestive health.

3. Include Prebiotic-Rich Foods:

- Include prebiotic-rich foods such as garlic, onions, leeks, asparagus, bananas, oats, and Jerusalem artichokes in your meals. These foods contain non-digestible fibers that serve as food for beneficial gut bacteria, helping to nourish and support their growth.

4. Focus on Whole, Unprocessed Foods:
   - Select whole, minimally processed foods over refined and highly processed ones. Whole foods are rich in nutrients, fiber, and antioxidants, while processed foods often contain added sugars, unhealthy fats, and artificial additives that can disrupt gut health.

5. Balance Macronutrients:
   - Aim for a balance of carbohydrates, proteins, and fats in each meal. Choose complex carbohydrates like whole grains and starchy vegetables, lean sources of protein such as poultry, fish, and legumes, and healthy fats like avocado, nuts, and olive oil.

6. Include Fermented Foods:
   - Incorporate fermented foods into your meal plan on a regular basis to support gut health. Experiment with different types of fermented foods, such as yogurt bowls topped with fruit and nuts, salads with homemade fermented vegetables, and stir-fries with tempeh or kimchi.

7. Stay Hydrated:
   - Throughout the day, sip on lots of water to stay hydrated and promote healthy digestion. Herbal teas, infused water with fruits or herbs, and coconut

water are also hydrating options that can contribute to gut health.

8. Plan Balanced Meals and Snacks:
   - Plan balanced meals and snacks that include a variety of nutrient-dense foods from all food groups. Aim for a combination of carbohydrates, proteins, and fats to provide sustained energy and support digestive health throughout the day.

9. Listen to Your Body:
   - Pay attention to how different foods make you feel and adjust your meal plan accordingly. Everyone's digestive system is unique, so it's important to listen to your body's cues and make choices that support your individual needs and preferences.

By incorporating these principles into your meal planning, you can create a gut-healthy diet that nourishes your body, supports digestive wellness, and promotes overall health and vitality. Experiment with different foods, flavors, and recipes to find what works best for you and enjoy the benefits of a thriving gut microbiome.

PLANNING MEALS AND SNACKS

Planning meals and snacks is an important aspect of maintaining a healthy diet and supporting digestive wellness. Here are some tips for effective meal and snack planning:

1. Set Aside Time for Planning:

- Dedicate a specific time each week to plan your meals and snacks. This could be on a weekend or whenever is most convenient for you. Planning ahead helps you make healthier choices and reduces the likelihood of resorting to unhealthy options when you're short on time.

2. Consider Your Schedule:

- Take into account your schedule for the upcoming week when planning meals and snacks. If you have busy days or evenings, opt for quick and easy meals that require minimal preparation. On days when you have more time, you can plan more elaborate meals or try out new recipes.

3. Plan Balanced Meals:

- Aim for a carbohydrate, protein, and fat balance in each meal. Choose whole, minimally processed foods from all food groups to provide a variety of nutrients and support overall health. Incorporate plenty of fruits, veggies, whole grains, lean proteins, and healthy fats into your diet plan.

4. Batch Cook and Prep Ingredients:

- Consider batch cooking and prepping ingredients in advance to save time during the week. Cook grains, beans, and proteins in large batches and portion them out for easy meals. Chop vegetables, wash fruits, and prepare snacks like homemade trail mix or yogurt parfaits to have on hand for quick and convenient options.

5. Mix and Match:

- Get creative with meal combinations and mix and match ingredients to keep things interesting. For example, use leftover roasted vegetables to top salads or add to grain bowls, or repurpose cooked chicken into wraps, sandwiches, or salads for a variety of meals throughout the week.

6. Pack Portable Snacks:

- Plan and pack portable snacks to have on hand when you're on the go. Choose nutrient-dense options like fresh fruit, vegetables with hummus or nut butter, Greek yogurt, hard-boiled eggs, nuts and seeds, whole grain crackers with cheese, or homemade energy bars.

7. Listen to Your Body:

- Pay attention to your hunger and fullness cues and adjust your meal and snack plan accordingly. Eat when you're hungry and stop when you're satisfied, rather than following a rigid schedule. Honor your cravings and preferences while making choices that support your health and well-being.

8. Stay Flexible:

- Be flexible with your meal and snack plan and don't be afraid to adapt as needed. If something comes up or you're not in the mood for what you had planned, switch things up and choose a different option. Remember that meal preparation is intended to make your life easier, not to cause stress.

By taking the time to plan meals and snacks ahead of time, you can make healthier choices, save time and money, and support your digestive wellness and overall health. Experiment with different recipes, flavors, and combinations to keep things exciting and enjoyable, and find a meal planning routine that works best for you.

SAMPLE MEAL PLANS FOR DIFFERENT LIFESTYLES

Certainly! Here are sample meal plans tailored for different lifestyles, incorporating principles of gut health and balanced nutrition:

1. **Busy Professional**

   Breakfast: Greek yogurt parfait with mixed berries, chia seeds, and a drizzle of honey.

   Lunch: Quinoa salad with mixed greens, roasted vegetables, chickpeas, avocado, and a lemon-tahini dressing.

   Snack: Sliced apple with almond butter.

Dinner: Grilled salmon with roasted sweet potatoes and steamed broccoli.

Snack: Carrot sticks with hummus.

2. **Fitness Enthusiast**

Breakfast: Protein smoothie with spinach, banana, protein powder, almond milk, and a tablespoon of ground flaxseed.

Mid-Morning Snack: Whole grain toast with mashed avocado and sliced hard-boiled egg.

Lunch: Quinoa and black bean bowl with mixed greens, grilled chicken, bell peppers, corn, and salsa.

Afternoon Snack: Greek yogurt with mixed berries and a sprinkle of granola.

Dinner: Stir-fried tofu with brown rice, broccoli, bell peppers, snap peas, and a ginger-soy sauce.

3. **On-the-Go Parent**

Breakfast: Overnight oats with almond milk, sliced banana, and a handful of chopped nuts.

Mid-Morning Snack: Apple slices with string cheese.

Lunch: Turkey and avocado wrap with whole grain tortilla, mixed greens, tomato, and mustard.

Afternoon Snack: Baby carrots with hummus.

Dinner: Baked chicken breasts with quinoa pilaf and roasted vegetables (e.g., carrots, Brussels sprouts, and cauliflower).

4. **Vegetarian/Vegan Lifestyle**

Breakfast: Tofu scramble with spinach, cherry tomatoes, onions, and whole grain toast.

Mid-Morning Snack: Sliced cucumber with tahini drizzle.

Lunch: Lentil soup with a side of mixed greens salad with chickpeas, roasted beets, and balsamic vinaigrette.

Afternoon Snack: Rice cakes with almond butter and sliced strawberries.

Dinner: Spaghetti squash with marinara sauce and sautéed mushrooms, served with a side of steamed green beans.

5. **Flexitarian (Occasional Meat Eater)**

Breakfast: Whole grain toast with smashed avocado, sliced tomatoes, and a fried egg.

Mid-Morning Snack: Mixed nuts and dried fruit trail mix.

Lunch: Quinoa and black bean stuffed bell peppers with a side of mixed greens salad.

Afternoon Snack: Cottage cheese with pineapple chunks.

Dinner: Grilled shrimp skewers with quinoa tabbouleh and roasted zucchini and bell peppers.

These sample meal plans provide a variety of nutrient-dense, balanced meals and snacks suitable for different lifestyles while promoting gut health and overall well-being. Feel free to adjust portion sizes and ingredients based on individual preferences and dietary needs.

TIPS FOR MEAL PREP AND GROCERY SHOPPING

Certainly! Here are some tips for meal prep and grocery shopping to help you stay organized, save time, and make healthier choices:

Meal Prep:

1. **Plan Ahead:** Take some time each week to plan your meals and snacks. Consider your schedule, dietary preferences, and nutritional needs when creating your meal plan.

2. **Batch Cooking:** Cook large batches of grains, proteins, and vegetables in advance to use in multiple meals throughout the week. Portion them out into containers for easy grab-and-go meals.

3. **Prep Ingredients:** Wash, chop, and prep fruits, vegetables, and other ingredients ahead of time. Store them in airtight containers or resealable bags in the refrigerator for quick and easy meal assembly.

4. **Use Mason Jars:** Mason jars are great for portioning out salads, overnight oats, and smoothie ingredients. Layer ingredients in the jars for easy grab-and-go meals or snacks.

5. **Invest in Meal Prep Containers:** Invest in a set of meal prep containers in various sizes to portion out meals and snacks for the week. Choose containers that are microwave and dishwasher safe for easy reheating and cleaning.

6. **Label and Date:** Label your meal prep containers with the contents and date of preparation to help you keep track of what's inside

and when it was made. This will help prevent food waste and ensure you're eating fresh meals.

Grocery Shopping:

1. **Make a List:** Before heading to the grocery store, make a list of the items you need based on your meal plan. Organize your list by categories such as produce, dairy, protein, grains, and pantry staples to streamline your shopping trip.

2. **Stick to the Perimeter:** Shop the perimeter of the grocery store where fresh produce, meat, dairy, and other whole foods are typically located. Limit your time in the center aisles where processed and packaged foods are found.

3. **Read Labels:** Take the time to read labels and ingredients lists when choosing packaged foods. Look for products with minimal ingredients, low added sugars, and minimal processing.

4. **Choose Seasonal Produce:** Opt for seasonal fruits and vegetables, as they tend to be fresher, more flavorful, and less expensive. Check out farmers' markets or local produce stands for a variety of seasonal options.

5. **Stock Up on Staples:** Keep your pantry stocked with staple ingredients such as whole grains, beans, canned tomatoes, herbs and spices, olive oil, vinegar, and nuts and seeds. These

ingredients form the foundation of many healthy meals and recipes.

6. **Shop with a Budget in Mind:** Set a budget for your grocery shopping trip and stick to it. Look for sales, use coupons, and consider buying store-brand items to save money without sacrificing quality.

By implementing these tips for meal prep and grocery shopping, you can streamline your meal planning process, make healthier food choices, and save time and money in the kitchen. With a little preparation and organization, you can set yourself up for success and enjoy delicious, nutritious meals throughout the week.

CHAPTER FOUR

GUT-HEALTHY RECIPES FOR WOMEN

Here are a few Gut health recipes tailored for women.

BREAKFAST IDEAS

1) Greek yogurt parfait with mixed berries, chia seeds, and a drizzle of honey.

Here's the recipe for a Greek yogurt parfait with mixed berries, chia seeds, and a drizzle of honey, along with detailed instructions, estimated cooking time, and nutritional value:

Ingredients:
- 1/2 cup Greek yogurt (plain, unsweetened)
- 1/4 cup of mixed berries, including blueberries, raspberries, and strawberries
- 1 tablespoon chia seeds
- 1 teaspoon honey (or to taste)

Instructions:
1. **Prepare Ingredients:** Wash and dry the mixed berries. If using strawberries, hull and slice them.

2. **Layer Yogurt:** In a glass or bowl, start by layering half of the Greek yogurt at the bottom.
3. **Add Berries:** Add half of the mixed berries on top of the yogurt layer.
4. **Sprinkle Chia Seeds:** Sprinkle half of the chia seeds over the berries.
5. **Repeat Layers:** Repeat the layers with the remaining Greek yogurt, mixed berries, and chia seeds.
6. **Drizzle Honey:** Drizzle honey evenly over the top of the parfait.
7. **Serve:** Serve immediately and enjoy this nutritious and delicious Greek yogurt parfait!

Cooking Time: 5 minutes (no cooking required)

Nutritional Value (per serving):
- Calories: 150
- Protein: 12g
- Carbohydrates: 18g
- Fat: 4g
- Fiber: 5g

This Greek yogurt parfait is packed with protein, fiber, and antioxidants from the Greek yogurt, mixed berries, and chia seeds. The drizzle of honey adds a touch of sweetness while still keeping the overall sugar content low. Enjoy this parfait for breakfast, as a snack, or even as a healthy dessert option!

2) Protein Smoothie

Here's a protein smoothie recipe along with detailed instructions, estimated preparation time, and nutritional value:

Green Protein Smoothie:

Ingredients:
- 1 cup spinach leaves
- 1/2 banana
- 1/2 cup frozen mango chunks
- 1 scoop vanilla protein powder
- 1 tablespoon chia seeds
- One cup of unsweetened almond milk, or any other preferred milk
- Ice cubes (optional)

Instructions:
1. **Prepare Ingredients:** Wash the spinach leaves and peel the banana. If not using pre-frozen mango chunks, peel and dice a ripe mango.
2. **Add Ingredients to Blender:** In a blender, add the spinach leaves, banana, frozen mango chunks, vanilla protein powder, chia seeds, and unsweetened almond milk.
3. **Blend Until Smooth:** Blend all the ingredients until smooth and creamy. If desired, add a few ice cubes for a colder and thicker consistency.
4. **Adjust Consistency:** If the smoothie is too thick, add more almond milk in small increments

until you reach your desired consistency. Add more frozen fruit or ice cubes if it's too thin.

5. **Serve:** Pour the smoothie into a glass and enjoy immediately for optimal freshness and taste!

Preparation Time: 5 minutes

Nutritional Value (per serving):
- **Calories:** 300
- **Protein:** 25g
- **Carbohydrates:** 35g
- **Fat:** 8g
- **Fiber:** 9g

This green protein smoothie is packed with nutrients, including protein, fiber, vitamins, and minerals. It's a refreshing and delicious way to fuel your body and keep you satisfied until your next meal or snack. Feel free to customize the recipe by adding other ingredients such as berries, nut butter, or Greek yogurt to suit your taste preferences and nutritional needs. Enjoy!

3) Overnight Oats With Berries And Almonds:

Here's a simple and delicious recipe for Overnight Oats with Berries and Almonds, along with detailed instructions, estimated preparation time, and nutritional value:

Ingredients:

- 1/2 cup rolled oats
- 1/2 cup unsweetened almond milk (or any milk of choice)
- 1/4 cup Greek yogurt (plain or vanilla)
- - A half cup of mixed berries, including raspberries, blueberries, and strawberries
- 1 tablespoon sliced almonds
- 1 teaspoon honey or maple syrup (optional, for sweetness)
- Pinch of cinnamon (optional)

Instructions:
1. **Combine Ingredients:** In a mason jar or airtight container, combine rolled oats, unsweetened almond milk, Greek yogurt, and a pinch of cinnamon if desired.
2. **Add Berries:** Add mixed berries on top of the oat mixture. You can either mix them in or layer them on top.
3. **Add Almonds:** Sprinkle sliced almonds on top of the berries.
4. **Sweeten (Optional):** If desired, drizzle honey or maple syrup over the oats for added sweetness.
5. **Mix and Refrigerate:** Stir all the ingredients together until well combined. Cover the jar or container with a lid and refrigerate overnight, or for at least 4 hours, to allow the oats to soften and absorb the liquid.
6. **Serve:** In the morning, give the overnight oats a good stir. You can enjoy them cold straight from the fridge or heat them in the microwave for a warm breakfast. Optionally, you can top with

additional fresh berries and almonds before serving.

Preparation Time: 5 minutes (plus overnight chilling)

Nutritional Value (per serving):
- **Calories:** 300
- **Protein:** 12g
- **Carbohydrates:** 40g
- **Fat:** 10g
- **Fiber:** 8g

This overnight oats recipe is a nutritious and convenient breakfast option that's packed with fiber, protein, healthy fats, and antioxidants from the oats, berries, and almonds. It's customizable to your taste preferences, so feel free to adjust the ingredients and sweetness level to suit your liking. Enjoy this delicious and satisfying breakfast to start your day on the right foot!

4) Tofu scramble with spinach, cherry tomatoes, onions, and whole grain toast.

Here's a delicious recipe for Tofu Scramble with Spinach, Cherry Tomatoes, Onions, and Whole Grain Toast, complete with detailed instructions, estimated preparation time, and nutritional value:

Ingredients:

- One firm tofu block that has been drained and
pressed
- One tablespoon of cooking oil, or olive oil of your
preference
- 1/2 onion, diced
- 1 cup cherry tomatoes, halved
- 2 cups fresh spinach leaves
- 2 cloves garlic, minced
- 1 teaspoon turmeric powder
- 1/2 teaspoon cumin powder
- Salt and pepper to taste
- Whole grain toast, for serving

Instructions:
1. **Prepare Tofu:** Drain the tofu and press it to
remove excess moisture. Use a tofu press or wrap
the tofu block in paper towels and place a heavy
object on top for about 15-20 minutes.
2. **Sauté Vegetables:** In a large skillet, heat
olive oil over medium heat. Add diced onion and
cook for 2-3 minutes until softened.
3. **Add Tomatoes and Spinach:** Add cherry
tomatoes to the skillet and cook for 2 minutes until
they start to soften. Then, add fresh spinach leaves
and minced garlic to the skillet. Cook for another
2-3 minutes until the spinach wilts.
4. **Crumble Tofu:** Crumble the pressed tofu into
the skillet using your hands or a fork. Break it into
small pieces resembling scrambled eggs.
5. **Season:** Sprinkle turmeric powder and cumin
powder over the tofu and vegetables. Season with

salt and pepper to taste. Stir well to combine and evenly distribute the spices.

6. **Cook:** Cook the tofu scramble for 5-7 minutes, stirring occasionally, until heated through and the flavors meld together.

7. **Toast Bread:** While the tofu scramble is cooking, toast the whole grain bread until golden brown and crispy.

8. **Serve:** Once the tofu scramble is cooked to your liking, remove it from the heat. Serve hot alongside whole grain toast.

9. **Enjoy:** Divide the tofu scramble and whole grain toast among serving plates. Serve immediately and enjoy this nutritious and satisfying breakfast!

Preparation Time: 20 minutes

Nutritional Value (per serving, including toast):
- **Calories:** 300
- **Protein:** 20g
- **Carbohydrates:** 25g
- **Fat:** 14g
- **Fiber:** 6g

This tofu scramble with spinach, cherry tomatoes, onions, and whole grain toast is a wholesome and satisfying breakfast option that's packed with protein, fiber, vitamins, and minerals. Enjoy it as a nutritious start to your day or any time you're craving a delicious and filling meal!

5) Whole grain toast with smashed avocado, sliced tomatoes, and a fried egg.

Here's a simple yet delicious recipe for Whole Grain Toast with Smashed Avocado, Sliced Tomatoes, and a Fried Egg, complete with detailed instructions, estimated preparation time, and nutritional value:

Ingredients:
- 2 slices whole grain bread, toasted
- 1 ripe avocado
- 1 small tomato, thinly sliced
- 2 eggs
- Salt and pepper to taste
- Optional toppings: red pepper flakes, fresh herbs (such as parsley or chives)

Instructions:
1. **Prepare Avocado:** Cut the ripe avocado in half and remove the pit. Scoop the avocado flesh into a small bowl. Use a fork to mash the avocado until smooth or slightly chunky, depending on your preference.
2. **Toast Bread:** Toast the slices of whole grain bread until golden brown and crispy.
3. **Fry Eggs:** In a non-stick skillet, heat a little cooking oil over medium heat. Crack the eggs into the skillet and cook for 2-3 minutes until the whites are set but the yolks are still runny. Season with salt and pepper to taste.

4. **Assemble:** Spread a generous amount of smashed avocado onto each slice of toasted bread. Arrange thinly sliced tomatoes on top of the avocado.
5. **Add Fried Egg:** Carefully place a fried egg on each slice of toast, on top of the avocado and tomatoes.
6. **Season:** Sprinkle the fried eggs with a little more salt and pepper if desired. Optionally, garnish with red pepper flakes or fresh herbs for added flavor and color.
7. **Serve:** Serve the whole grain toast with smashed avocado, sliced tomatoes, and a fried egg immediately while still warm.

Preparation Time: 10 minutes

Nutritional Value (per serving, including two slices of toast and two eggs):
- **Calories:** 400
- **Protein:** 17g
- **Carbohydrates:** 30g
- **Fat:** 25g
- **Fiber:** 10g

This Whole Grain Toast with Smashed Avocado, Sliced Tomatoes, and a Fried Egg is a satisfying and nutritious breakfast option that's packed with protein, healthy fats, and fiber. Enjoy it as a hearty breakfast or brunch, or any time you're craving a delicious and wholesome meal!

LUNCH RECIPES

The following are some lunch recipes with detailed instructions.

1) Quinoa salad with mixed greens, roasted vegetables, chickpeas, avocado, and a lemon-tahini dressing

Here's a delicious recipe for Quinoa Salad with Mixed Greens, Roasted Vegetables, Chickpeas, Avocado, and a Lemon-Tahini Dressing, complete with detailed instructions, estimated preparation time, and nutritional value:

Ingredients:

For the Salad:
- 1 cup quinoa, rinsed
- 2 cups mixed greens (such as spinach, arugula, or kale)
- 1 cup roasted vegetables (such as sweet potatoes, bell peppers, and zucchini)
- 1 can chickpeas, drained and rinsed
- 1 ripe avocado, diced

For the Lemon-Tahini Dressing:
- 1/4 cup tahini
- Juice of 1 lemon
- 2 tablespoons olive oil
- 1 clove garlic, minced

- Salt and pepper to taste
- Water (as needed to thin the dressing)

Instructions:

1. **Cook Quinoa:** In a medium saucepan, combine 1 cup of quinoa with 2 cups of water. Bring to a boil, then lower the heat, cover, and cook for 15 to 20 minutes, or until the quinoa is fluffy and soft. After removing from the heat source, let it cool.

2. **Prepare Roasted Vegetables:** Preheat your oven to 400°F (200°C). Toss your choice of vegetables (such as sweet potatoes, bell peppers, and zucchini) with olive oil, salt, and pepper. Spread them out on a baking sheet in a single layer and roast for 20-25 minutes, or until they are tender and slightly caramelized. Let them cool slightly.

3. **Make Lemon-Tahini Dressing:** In a small bowl, whisk together tahini, lemon juice, olive oil, minced garlic, salt, and pepper until smooth. If the dressing is too thick, you can thin it out with a little water until you reach your desired consistency.

4. **Assemble Salad:** In a large mixing bowl, combine cooked quinoa, mixed greens, roasted vegetables, chickpeas, and diced avocado.

5. **Add Dressing:** Drizzle the lemon-tahini dressing over the salad and toss gently to coat everything evenly.

6. **Serve:** Transfer the quinoa salad to serving plates or bowls. You can garnish with additional toppings like fresh herbs or toasted nuts if desired.

Preparation Time: 30 minutes

Nutritional Value (per serving):
- **Calories:** 400
- **Protein:** 12g
- **Carbohydrates:** 40g
- **Fat:** 20g
- **Fiber:** 10g

This Quinoa Salad with Mixed Greens, Roasted Vegetables, Chickpeas, Avocado, and Lemon-Tahini Dressing is a nutritious and satisfying meal packed with protein, healthy fats, fiber, and vitamins. It's perfect for lunch or as a light dinner option. Enjoy!

2) Turkey and avocado wrap with whole grain tortilla, mixed greens, tomato, and mustard.

Here's a delicious recipe for a Turkey and Avocado Wrap with Whole Grain Tortilla, Mixed Greens, Tomato, and Mustard, complete with detailed instructions, estimated preparation time, and nutritional value:

Turkey and Avocado Wrap:

Ingredients:
- 1 whole grain tortilla
- 2-3 slices of turkey breast
- 1/4 avocado, sliced
- Handful of mixed greens
- 1 small tomato, thinly sliced
- One tablespoon of whole grain or Dijon mustard
- Salt and pepper to taste

Instructions:

1. **Prepare Ingredients:** Lay the whole grain tortilla flat on a clean surface. Slice the turkey breast, avocado, and tomato thinly.

2. **Assemble Wrap:** Spread the mustard evenly over the tortilla, leaving about 1-inch border around the edges. Layer the sliced turkey breast, avocado slices, mixed greens, and tomato slices on top of the mustard.

3. **Season:** Season with salt and pepper to taste.

4. **Wrap:** Starting from one edge, tightly roll the tortilla around the filling ingredients, tucking in the sides as you go to prevent the filling from spilling out.

5. **Slice (Optional):** If desired, you can slice the wrap in half diagonally for easier eating or leave it whole.

6. **Serve:** Serve the turkey and avocado wrap immediately or wrap it in parchment paper or foil for an on-the-go meal.

****Preparation Time:**** 10 minutes

****Nutritional Value (per serving):****
- **Calories:** 300
- **Protein:** 20g
- **Carbohydrates:** 25g
- **Fat:** 15g
- **Fiber:** 8g

This Turkey and Avocado Wrap with Whole Grain Tortilla, Mixed Greens, Tomato, and Mustard is a balanced and satisfying meal that provides protein, healthy fats, fiber, and essential nutrients. Enjoy it for lunch or a quick and nutritious snack!

3) Lentil soup with a side of mixed greens salad with chickpeas, roasted beets, and balsamic vinaigrette.

Here's a delicious recipe for Lentil Soup with a Side of Mixed Greens Salad with Chickpeas, Roasted Beets, and Balsamic Vinaigrette, complete with detailed instructions, estimated preparation time, and nutritional value:

Lentil Soup:

Ingredients:
- One cup of washed and drained dried green lentils
- 1 onion, diced
- 2 carrots, diced
- 2 celery stalks, diced
- 3 cloves garlic, minced
- 1 can (14 oz) diced tomatoes
- 4 cups vegetable broth
- 1 teaspoon ground cumin
- 1 teaspoon ground coriander
- 1/2 teaspoon smoked paprika
- Salt and pepper to taste
- Fresh parsley or cilantro for garnish (optional)

Instructions:

1. **Cook Lentils:** In a large pot, heat some olive oil over medium heat. Add diced onion, carrots, and celery. Cook, stirring occasionally, for about 5 minutes until the vegetables start to soften.

2. **Add Garlic and Spices:** Add minced garlic, ground cumin, ground coriander, and smoked paprika to the pot. Cook for another minute until fragrant.

3. **Add Lentils and Tomatoes:** Add rinsed and drained lentils and diced tomatoes (with their juices) to the pot. Stir to combine.

4. **Simmer:** Pour in vegetable broth and bring the soup to a simmer. Reduce heat to low, cover, and let it simmer for about 20-25 minutes until the lentils are tender.

5. **Season:** Season the soup with salt and pepper to taste. Adjust the seasoning as needed.

6. **Serve:** Ladle the lentil soup into bowls. Garnish with fresh parsley or cilantro if desired.

Preparation Time: 40 minutes

Nutritional Value (per serving):
- **Calories:** 250
- **Protein:** 15g
- **Carbohydrates:** 45g
- **Fat:** 2g
- **Fiber:** 12g

4)**Mixed Greens Salad with Chickpeas, Roasted Beets, and Balsamic Vinaigrette:**

Ingredients:
- Four cups of mixed greens, including romaine, spinach, and arugula
 - One 14-oz can of washed and drained chickpeas
- 2 medium-sized roasted beets, diced

- 1/4 cup balsamic vinaigrette dressing

Instructions:

1. **Prepare Salad:** In a large bowl, toss together mixed greens, drained and rinsed chickpeas, and diced roasted beets.

2. **Dress Salad:** Drizzle balsamic vinaigrette dressing over the salad. To uniformly coat all the ingredients, lightly toss.

3. **Serve:** Divide the mixed greens salad among serving plates.

Preparation Time: 15 minutes

Nutritional Value (per serving):
- **Calories:** 200
- **Protein:** 10g
- **Carbohydrates:** 30g
- **Fat:** 6g
- **Fiber:** 8g

This Lentil Soup with a Side of Mixed Greens Salad with Chickpeas, Roasted Beets, and Balsamic Vinaigrette is a hearty and nutritious meal that's packed with protein, fiber, vitamins, and minerals. Enjoy it for a satisfying lunch or dinner!

DINNER RECIPES

The following are some dinner recipes with detailed instructions:

1) Grilled salmon with roasted sweet potatoes and steamed broccoli.

Here's a delicious and nutritious recipe for Grilled Salmon with Roasted Sweet Potatoes and Steamed Broccoli, complete with detailed instructions, estimated preparation time, and nutritional value:

Grilled Salmon:

Ingredients:
- 2 salmon fillets (6-8 oz each), skin-on
- 1 tablespoon olive oil
- 1 teaspoon lemon zest
- 1 tablespoon lemon juice
- 2 cloves garlic, minced
- Salt and pepper to taste
- Fresh herbs (like dill or parsley) for garnish

Instructions:

1. **Prepare Salmon Marinade:** In a small bowl, whisk together olive oil, lemon zest, lemon juice, minced garlic, salt, and pepper to create the marinade.

2. **Marinate Salmon:** Place the salmon fillets in a shallow dish or resealable plastic bag. Pour the marinade over the salmon, making sure it's evenly coated. Allow the salmon to marinate in the refrigerator for at least 30 minutes, or up to 2 hours for maximum flavor.

3. **Preheat Grill:** Preheat your grill to medium-high heat (around 400°F or 200°C). To keep the grill grates from sticking, lightly oil them.

4. **Grill Salmon:** Remove the salmon fillets from the marinade and shake off any excess. With the skin side facing down, place the salmon fillets onto the heated grill.. Grill for 4-5 minutes per side, or until the salmon is cooked through and easily flakes with a fork. To keep the salmon moist and tender, don't overcook it.

5. **Serve:** Once the salmon is cooked, remove it from the grill and transfer it to serving plates. Garnish with fresh herbs, if desired.

Preparation Time: 10 minutes (plus marinating time)

Nutritional Value (per serving):
- **Calories:** 300
- **Protein:** 30g
- **Carbohydrates:** 0g
- **Fat:** 20g

- **Fiber:** 0g

Roasted Sweet Potatoes:

Ingredients:
- 2 medium sweet potatoes, peeled and diced
- 1 tablespoon olive oil
- 1 teaspoon smoked paprika
- Salt and pepper to taste

Instructions:

1. **Preheat Oven:** Preheat your oven to 400°F (200°C). For easier cleanup, line a baking pan with aluminum foil or parchment paper.

2. **Prepare Sweet Potatoes:** In a large bowl, toss the diced sweet potatoes with olive oil, smoked paprika, salt, and pepper until evenly coated.

3. **Roast Sweet Potatoes:** Spread the seasoned sweet potatoes out in a single layer on the prepared baking sheet. Roast in the preheated oven for 25-30 minutes, flipping halfway through, until they are tender and caramelized.

4. **Serve:** Once the sweet potatoes are roasted to perfection, remove them from the oven and transfer them to serving plates.

Preparation Time: 10 minutes

Nutritional Value (per serving):
- **Calories:** 150
- **Protein:** 2g
- **Carbohydrates:** 25g
- **Fat:** 5g
- **Fiber:** 4g

Steamed Broccoli:

Ingredients:
- 2 cups broccoli florets
- Water for steaming
- Salt to taste (optional)

Instructions:

1. **Steam Broccoli:** Fill a pot with about an inch of water and place a steamer basket inside.Over medium-high heat, bring the water to a boil.

2. Add the broccoli florets to the steamer basket, cover the pot, and steam for 4-5 minutes, or until the broccoli is bright green and tender-crisp.

3. **Season:** Once the broccoli is steamed, remove it from the heat and transfer it to a serving dish. If preferred, add a little salt for seasoning.

4. **Serve:** Serve the steamed broccoli alongside the grilled salmon and roasted sweet potatoes.

Preparation Time: 5 minutes

Nutritional Value (per serving):
- **Calories:** 30
- **Protein:** 3g
- **Carbohydrates:** 6g
- **Fat:** 0g
- **Fiber:** 3g

This Grilled Salmon with Roasted Sweet Potatoes and Steamed Broccoli is a balanced and satisfying meal that's rich in protein, healthy fats, fiber, vitamins, and minerals. Enjoy this nutritious dish for a flavorful and wholesome dinner!

2) Stir-fried tofu with brown rice, broccoli, bell peppers, snap peas, and a ginger-soy sauce.

Here's a flavorful recipe for Stir-Fried Tofu with Brown Rice, Broccoli, Bell Peppers, Snap Peas, and a Ginger-Soy Sauce, complete with detailed instructions, estimated preparation time, and nutritional value:

Stir-Fried Tofu with Brown Rice:

Ingredients:

For the Stir-Fry:
- 1 block firm tofu, pressed and cubed
- 2 cups cooked brown rice

- 1 cup broccoli florets
- 1 bell pepper, thinly sliced
- 1 cup snap peas, trimmed
- 2 cloves garlic, minced
- 1 tablespoon ginger, minced
- 2 tablespoons sesame oil (divided)
- Salt and pepper to taste
- Sesame seeds for garnish (optional)
- Chopped green onions for garnish (optional)

For the Ginger-Soy Sauce:

- Three tablespoons of soy sauce (or tamari for gluten-free).
- 1 tablespoon rice vinegar
- 1 tablespoon maple syrup or honey
- 1 teaspoon sesame oil
- 1 teaspoon fresh ginger, grated
- 1 teaspoon cornstarch (optional, for thickening)

Instructions:

1. **Prepare Tofu:** Press the tofu to remove excess moisture by wrapping it in paper towels and placing a heavy object on top for about 15-20 minutes. Then, cut the tofu into cubes.

2. **Cook Brown Rice:** Prepare brown rice according to package instructions and set aside.

3. **Make Ginger-Soy Sauce:** In a small bowl, whisk together soy sauce, rice vinegar, maple syrup

or honey, sesame oil, and grated ginger. If you prefer a thicker sauce, you can dissolve cornstarch in a tablespoon of water and add it to the sauce. Set aside.

4. **Stir-Fry Tofu:** Heat one tablespoon of sesame oil in a large skillet or wok over medium-high heat. Add the cubed tofu and cook for 5-7 minutes, stirring occasionally, until golden brown and crispy on all sides. Take out and place aside the tofu from the skillet.

5. **Stir-Fry Vegetables:** In the same skillet, heat the remaining tablespoon of sesame oil over medium-high heat. Add the chopped ginger and garlic, and heat for one minute, or until fragrant. Add broccoli florets, sliced bell pepper, and snap peas to the skillet. Stir-fry for 5-7 minutes until the vegetables are tender-crisp.

6. **Combine Tofu and Vegetables:** Return the cooked tofu to the skillet with the vegetables. Pour the ginger-soy sauce over the tofu and vegetables, stirring to coat evenly. Cook for an additional 2-3 minutes until heated through and the sauce thickens slightly.

7. **Serve:** Serve the stir-fried tofu and vegetables over cooked brown rice. If desired, garnish with sesame seeds and chopped green onions

Preparation Time: 30 minutes

Nutritional Value (per serving):
- **Calories:** 350
- **Protein:** 15g
- **Carbohydrates:** 45g
- **Fat:** 12g
- **Fiber:** 8g

This Stir-Fried Tofu with Brown Rice, Broccoli, Bell Peppers, Snap Peas, and Ginger-Soy Sauce is a delicious and nutritious plant-based meal that's packed with protein, fiber, vitamins, and minerals. Enjoy this flavorful dish for a satisfying lunch or dinner!

3) Baked chicken breasts with quinoa pilaf and roasted vegetables

Here's a delightful recipe for Baked Chicken Breasts with Quinoa Pilaf and Roasted Vegetables, complete with detailed instructions, estimated preparation time, and nutritional value:

Baked Chicken Breasts:

Ingredients:
- 2 boneless, skinless chicken breasts
- 1 tablespoon olive oil
- 1 teaspoon garlic powder
- 1 teaspoon paprika
- Salt and pepper to taste

Instructions:

1. **Preheat Oven:** Preheat your oven to 375°F (190°C). Either lightly spray cooking spray on a baking dish or line it with parchment paper.

2. **Prepare Chicken:** Use paper towels to pat the chicken breasts dry. Coat the chicken breast in olive oil on both sides.

3. **Season Chicken:** In a small bowl, mix together garlic powder, paprika, salt, and pepper. Rub the seasoning mixture evenly over both sides of the chicken breasts.

4. **Bake Chicken:** Place the seasoned chicken breasts in the prepared baking dish. Bake for 25 to 30 minutes, or until the chicken is cooked through and the internal temperature reaches 165°F (75°C), in a preheated oven.

5. **Rest and Serve:** Once the chicken is cooked, remove it from the oven and let it rest for a few minutes before slicing. Serve hot with quinoa pilaf and roasted vegetables.

Preparation Time: 35 minutes

Nutritional Value (per serving):
- **Calories:** 250
- **Protein:** 30g

- **Carbohydrates:** 0g
- **Fat:** 12g
- **Fiber:** 0g

Quinoa Pilaf:

Ingredients:
- 1 cup quinoa, rinsed and drained
- 2 cups chicken or vegetable broth
- 1 tablespoon olive oil
- 1 small onion, diced
- 2 cloves garlic, minced
- 1/2 cup diced carrots
- 1/2 cup diced bell peppers
- Salt and pepper to taste
- For garnish, use fresh cilantro or parsley (optional).

Instructions:

1. **Cook Quinoa:** Olive oil should be heated over medium heat in a medium saucepan. Add diced onion and garlic, and cook for 2-3 minutes until softened.

2. **Add Vegetables:** Add diced carrots and bell peppers to the saucepan. Cook for another 3-4 minutes until the vegetables are tender.

3. **Toast Quinoa:** Add rinsed and drained quinoa to the saucepan. Cook, stirring frequently, for 1-2 minutes to toast the quinoa.

4. **Simmer:** Pour chicken or vegetable broth into the saucepan. Bring the mixture to a boil, then reduce heat to low, cover, and let it simmer for 15-20 minutes, or until the quinoa is cooked and fluffy.

5. **Season:** Season the quinoa pilaf with salt and pepper to taste. Fluff it with a fork and garnish with fresh parsley or cilantro, if desired.

Preparation Time: 30 minutes

Nutritional Value (per serving):
- **Calories:** 200
- **Protein:** 5g
- **Carbohydrates:** 30g
- **Fat:** 8g
- **Fiber:** 4g

Roasted Vegetables:

Ingredients:
- 2 cups mixed vegetables (such as carrots, bell peppers, zucchini, and broccoli), chopped
- 1 tablespoon olive oil
- Salt and pepper to taste
- Optional seasonings: garlic powder, onion powder, dried herbs

Instructions:

1. **Preheat Oven:** Preheat your oven to 400°F (200°C). For easier cleanup, line a baking pan with aluminum foil or parchment paper.

2. **Prepare Vegetables:** In a large bowl, toss chopped mixed vegetables with olive oil, salt, pepper, and any desired seasonings until evenly coated.

3. **Roast Vegetables:** Spread the seasoned vegetables out in a single layer on the prepared baking sheet. Roast the vegetables in the preheated oven for 20 to 25 minutes, stirring occasionally, or until they are soft and caramelized.

4. **Serve:** Once the vegetables are roasted to perfection, remove them from the oven and serve alongside the baked chicken breasts and quinoa pilaf.

Preparation Time: 25 minutes

Nutritional Value (per serving):
- **Calories:** 100
- **Protein:** 2g
- **Carbohydrates:** 10g
- **Fat:** 6g
- **Fiber:** 4g

This Baked Chicken Breasts with Quinoa Pilaf and Roasted Vegetables is a wholesome and satisfying meal that's packed with protein, fiber, vitamins, and minerals. Enjoy this delicious and nutritious dish for a flavorful dinner!

4) Spaghetti squash with marinara sauce and sautéed mushrooms, served with a side of steamed green beans.

Here's a tasty and healthy recipe for Spaghetti Squash with Marinara Sauce and Sautéed Mushrooms, served with a side of Steamed Green Beans, complete with detailed instructions, estimated preparation time, and nutritional value:

Spaghetti Squash with Marinara Sauce and Sautéed Mushrooms:

Ingredients:

For the Spaghetti Squash:
- 1 medium spaghetti squash
- 1 tablespoon olive oil
- Salt and pepper to taste

For the Marinara Sauce:
- Two cups marinara sauce (store-bought or homemade)

For the Sautéed Mushrooms:
- 2 cups sliced mushrooms
- 2 cloves garlic, minced
- 1 tablespoon olive oil

- Salt and pepper to taste
- Fresh parsley for garnish (optional)

Instructions:

1. **Prepare Spaghetti Squash:** Preheat your oven to 400°F (200°C). Scoop out the seeds after cutting the spaghetti squash in half lengthwise. After applying some olive oil to the sliced sides, season with salt and pepper. Place the squash halves, cut side down, on a baking sheet lined with parchment paper. Bake in the preheated oven for 40-45 minutes, or until the squash is tender and easily pierced with a fork.

2. **Make Marinara Sauce:** While the spaghetti squash is baking, heat the marinara sauce in a saucepan over medium heat until heated through. Keep warm until ready to serve.

3. **Sauté Mushrooms:** In a large skillet, heat olive oil over medium heat. Add sliced mushrooms and minced garlic to the skillet. The mushrooms should be sautéed for 5 to 7 minutes, stirring periodically, until they are soft and golden brown. Season with salt and pepper to taste. Remove from heat and set aside.

4. **Scrape Spaghetti Squash:** Once the spaghetti squash is cooked, remove it from the oven and let it cool slightly. Using a fork, scrape the squash flesh into "spaghetti" strands.

5. **Assemble Dish:** Divide the spaghetti squash
strands among serving plates. Top each portion
with marinara sauce and sautéed mushrooms.
Garnish with fresh parsley, if desired.

Preparation Time: 50 minutes

Nutritional Value (per serving):
- **Calories:** 200
- **Protein:** 5g
- **Carbohydrates:** 35g
- **Fat:** 8g
- **Fiber:** 10g

Steamed Green Beans:

Ingredients:
- 2 cups green beans, trimmed
- Water for steaming
- Salt and pepper to taste
- Lemon wedges for serving (optional)

Instructions:

1. **Steam Green Beans:** Fill a pot with about an
inch of water and place a steamer basket inside.
Over medium-high heat, bring the water to a boil.
Add trimmed green beans to the steamer basket,
cover the pot, and steam for 4-5 minutes, or until
the green beans are bright green and tender-crisp.

2. **Season:** Once the green beans are steamed, remove them from the heat and transfer them to a serving dish. Season with salt and pepper to taste. Optional: serve with lemon wedges on the side.

Preparation Time: 10 minutes

Nutritional Value (per serving):
- **Calories:** 30
- **Protein:** 2g
- **Carbohydrates:** 6g
- **Fat:** 0g
- **Fiber:** 4g

This Spaghetti Squash with Marinara Sauce and Sautéed Mushrooms, served with Steamed Green Beans, is a flavorful and nutritious meal that's low in calories and packed with fiber, vitamins, and minerals. Enjoy this satisfying dish for a delicious dinner!

SNACKS AND DESSERTS

Certainly! Here are five snack and dessert recipes with detailed instructions, cooking time, and nutritional value:

1. **Greek Yogurt Parfait with Granola and mixed berries:**

Ingredients:

- 1 cup Greek yogurt
- half cup of mixed berries, including raspberries, blueberries, and strawberries
- 1/4 cup granola
- You can optionally drizzle with honey or maple syrup.

Instructions:
1. In a serving glass or bowl, layer Greek yogurt, mixed berries, and granola.
2. Repeat the layers until the glass or bowl is filled.
3. Drizzle honey or maple syrup on top, if desired.
4. Serve immediately and enjoy!

Preparation Time: 5 minutes

Nutritional Value (per serving):
- **Calories:** 250
- **Protein:** 18g
- **Carbohydrates:** 30g
- **Fat:** 8g
- **Fiber:** 4g

2. **Apple Slices with Peanut Butter and Dark Chocolate Chips:**

Ingredients:
- 1 apple, sliced
- 2 tablespoons peanut butter
- 1 tablespoon dark chocolate chips

Instructions:

1. Arrange apple slices on a plate.
2. Spread peanut butter on each apple slice.
3. Sprinkle dark chocolate chips on top.
4. Serve as a delicious and satisfying snack.

Preparation Time: 5 minutes

Nutritional Value (per serving):
- **Calories:** 250
- **Protein:** 6g
- **Carbohydrates:** 25g
- **Fat:** 15g
- **Fiber:** 5g

3. **Energy Bites with Oats, Peanut Butter, and Honey:**

Ingredients:
- 1 cup rolled oats
- 1/2 cup peanut butter
- 1/4 cup honey
- 1/4 cup dark chocolate chips
- 1/4 cup shredded coconut (optional)

Instructions:
1. In a mixing bowl, combine rolled oats, peanut butter, honey, dark chocolate chips, and shredded coconut (if using).
2. Stir until well combined.
3. With your hands, roll the mixture into little balls.
4. Place the energy bites on a baking sheet lined with parchment paper.

5. Before serving, let the food cool for at least half an hour in the refrigerator.
6. Enjoy these nutritious and energy-packed bites as a snack.

Preparation Time: 10 minutes (+ chilling time)

Nutritional Value (per serving, about 2 bites):
- **Calories:** 200
- **Protein:** 6g
- **Carbohydrates:** 20g
- **Fat:** 12g
- **Fiber:** 3g

4. **Frozen Banana Bites with Almond Butter and Dark Chocolate:**

Ingredients:
- two bananas, peeled and cut into slices
- 1/4 cup almond butter
- 1/4 cup dark chocolate chips

Instructions:
1. Arrange banana slices on a baking sheet lined with parchment paper.
2. Spread almond butter on half of the banana slices.
3. Top each almond butter-covered slice with another banana slice to create sandwiches.
4. Melt dark chocolate chips in the microwave or using a double boiler.

5. Dip each banana sandwich into the melted chocolate, coating it halfway.
6. Place the chocolate-covered banana bites back on the baking sheet.
7. Freeze for at least 1 hour until the chocolate is set.
8. Serve as a delicious frozen treat.

Preparation Time: 15 minutes (+ freezing time)

Nutritional Value (per serving, about 4 banana bites):
- **Calories:** 180
- **Protein:** 4g
- **Carbohydrates:** 25g
- **Fat:** 8g
- **Fiber:** 4g

5. **Chia Seed Pudding with Mango and Coconut Flakes:**

Ingredients:
- 1/4 cup chia seeds
- 1 cup coconut milk
- 1 tablespoon honey or maple syrup
- 1/2 teaspoon vanilla extract
- 1 ripe mango, diced
- 2 tablespoons unsweetened coconut flakes

Instructions:

1. In a mixing bowl, combine chia seeds, coconut milk, honey or maple syrup, and vanilla extract. Stir well.
2. Cover the bowl and refrigerate for at least 2 hours or overnight, allowing the chia seeds to absorb the liquid and thicken.
3. Once the chia pudding is set, divide it into serving cups or bowls.
4. Top each serving with diced mango and a sprinkle of unsweetened coconut flakes.
5. Serve chilled as a refreshing and nutritious dessert or snack.

Preparation Time: 5 minutes (+ chilling time)

Nutritional Value (per serving):
- **Calories:** 250
- **Protein:** 5g
- **Carbohydrates:** 30g
- **Fat:** 15g
- **Fiber:** 10g

Enjoy these delicious and nutritious snack and dessert recipes!

SMOOTHIES AND BEVERAGES

Sure! Here are five smoothie and beverage recipes with detailed instructions, preparation time, and nutritional value:

1. **Green Smoothie with Spinach, Banana, and Almond Milk:**

Ingredients:
- 1 ripe banana
- 1 cup fresh spinach leaves
- 1/2 cup almond milk
- 1 tablespoon honey or maple syrup (optional)
- Ice cubes (optional)

Instructions:
1. Place all ingredients in a blender.
2. Blend until smooth and creamy.
3. Taste and adjust sweetness, if desired, by adding honey or maple syrup.
4. If a colder smoothie is desired, add ice cubes and blend again until smooth.
5. Pour into glasses and enjoy immediately.

Preparation Time: 5 minutes

Nutritional Value (per serving):
- **Calories:** 150
- **Protein:** 3g
- **Carbohydrates:** 30g
- **Fat:** 2g
- **Fiber:** 5g

2. **Berry Blast Smoothie with Mixed Berries and Greek Yogurt:**

Ingredients:
- half cup of mixed berries, including raspberries, blueberries, and strawberries
- 1/2 cup Greek yogurt
- 1/2 cup almond milk
- 1 tablespoon honey or maple syrup (optional)
- Ice cubes (optional)

Instructions:
1. Place all ingredients in a blender.
2. Blend until smooth and well combined.
3. Taste and adjust sweetness, if desired, by adding honey or maple syrup.
4. Add ice cubes if a colder smoothie is preferred, and blend again until smooth.
5. Pour into glasses and serve immediately.

Preparation Time: 5 minutes

Nutritional Value (per serving):
- **Calories:** 200
- **Protein:** 10g
- **Carbohydrates:** 25g
- **Fat:** 5g
- **Fiber:** 6g

3. **Tropical Mango-Pineapple Smoothie with Coconut Water:**

Ingredients:
- 1 ripe mango, peeled and diced
- 1 cup fresh pineapple chunks

- 1/2 cup coconut water
- Juice of 1/2 lime
- 1 tablespoon honey or maple syrup (optional)
- Ice cubes (optional)

Instructions:
1. Place all ingredients in a blender.
2. Blend until smooth and creamy.
3. Taste and adjust sweetness, if desired, by adding honey or maple syrup.
4. For a colder smoothie, add ice cubes and blend again until smooth.
5. Pour into glasses and serve immediately, garnished with a slice of lime if desired.

Preparation Time: 5 minutes

Nutritional Value (per serving):
- **Calories:** 180
- **Protein:** 2g
- **Carbohydrates:** 40g
- **Fat:** 1g
- **Fiber:** 5g

4. **Banana-Oatmeal Smoothie with Peanut Butter and Honey:**

Ingredients:
- 1 ripe banana
- 1/4 cup rolled oats
- 1 tablespoon peanut butter
- 1 cup almond milk

- 1 tablespoon honey or maple syrup (optional)
- Ice cubes (optional)

Instructions:
1. Place all ingredients in a blender.
2. Blend until smooth and creamy.
3. Taste and adjust sweetness, if desired, by adding honey or maple syrup.
4. If a colder smoothie is preferred, add ice cubes and blend again until smooth.
5. Pour into glasses and enjoy immediately.

Preparation Time: 5 minutes

Nutritional Value (per serving):
- **Calories:** 250
- **Protein:** 7g
- **Carbohydrates:** 40g
- **Fat:** 8g
- **Fiber:** 6g

5. **Refreshing Cucumber-Mint Lemonade:**

Ingredients:
- 2 cucumbers, peeled and sliced
- Juice of 2 lemons
- 1/4 cup fresh mint leaves
- 4 cups water
- 2 tablespoons honey or maple syrup (optional)
- Ice cubes
- Sliced lemon and mint leaves for garnish

Instructions:
1. Place sliced cucumbers, lemon juice, mint leaves, and water in a blender.
2. Blend until smooth.
3. Strain the mixture through a fine mesh sieve to remove any solids.
4. Stir in honey or maple syrup, if desired, until sweetened to taste.
5. Before serving, let it cool for at least an hour in the refrigerator.
6. Serve over ice cubes, garnished with sliced lemon and mint leaves.

Preparation Time: 10 minutes (+ chilling time)

Nutritional Value (per serving):
- **Calories:** 50
- **Protein:** 1g
- **Carbohydrates:** 15g
- **Fat:** 0g
- **Fiber:** 2g

Enjoy these delicious and refreshing smoothie and beverage recipes!

CHAPTER FIVE

LIFESTYLES FACTORS FOR GUT HEALTH

Maintaining a healthy gut involves more than just diet; lifestyle factors also play a crucial role in supporting gut health. Here are several lifestyle factors that can positively impact gut health:

1. **Regular Exercise:** Physical activity promotes better digestion and can help regulate bowel movements. Exercise also supports a healthy balance of gut bacteria, contributing to overall gut health.

2. **Adequate Sleep:** Quality sleep is essential for gut health as it allows the body to repair and regenerate tissues, including the gut lining. Poor sleep habits can disrupt the gut microbiome and increase inflammation in the body.

3. **Stress Management:** Chronic stress can negatively impact gut health by altering gut motility, increasing inflammation, and disrupting the balance of gut bacteria. Practices such as mindfulness, meditation, yoga, and deep breathing exercises can help manage stress and promote gut health.

4. **Hydration:** Drinking enough water is vital for maintaining proper digestion and preventing constipation. Water helps flush toxins out of the body and supports the mucosal lining of the intestines, promoting a healthy gut environment.

5. **Limiting Alcohol and Caffeine:** Excessive alcohol consumption and high caffeine intake can disrupt the balance of gut bacteria and lead to inflammation in the gut. Moderation is key to maintaining gut health.

6. **Avoiding Smoking:** Smoking can have detrimental effects on gut health by disrupting the balance of gut bacteria and increasing the risk of inflammatory bowel diseases such as Crohn's disease and ulcerative colitis. Quitting smoking or avoiding exposure to secondhand smoke is essential for gut health.

7. **Maintaining a Healthy Weight:** Obesity and excess body fat can increase the risk of gut-related conditions such as acid reflux, gastroesophageal reflux disease (GERD), and inflammatory bowel diseases. Maintaining a healthy weight through a balanced diet and regular exercise can support gut health.

8. **Limiting Antibiotic Use:** Antibiotics can disrupt the balance of gut bacteria, leading to dysbiosis and increased susceptibility to gastrointestinal infections. Whenever possible, it's

essential to use antibiotics judiciously and only when necessary to minimize their impact on gut health.

By incorporating these lifestyle factors into daily routines, individuals can support a healthy gut microbiome and promote overall digestive wellness.

STRESS MANAGEMENT TECHNIQUES

Stress management is essential for maintaining overall well-being, including gut health. Here are several effective stress management techniques that can help reduce stress levels:

1. **Mindfulness Meditation:** Mindfulness meditation involves focusing on the present moment without judgment. Practicing mindfulness meditation regularly can help reduce stress, promote relaxation, and improve overall emotional well-being. Apps like Headspace and Calm offer guided mindfulness meditation sessions for beginners.

2. **Deep Breathing Exercises:** Deep breathing exercises, such as diaphragmatic breathing or belly breathing, can help activate the body's relaxation response and reduce stress levels. Practice deep breathing by Taking deep breaths through your

nose, stretch your abdomen, and then slowly exhale through your mouth.

3. **Progressive Muscle Relaxation (PMR):** PMR is a technique that involves tensing and relaxing different muscle groups in the body to promote relaxation. Starting from your toes and working your way up to your head, tense each muscle group for a few seconds and then release the tension, focusing on the sensation of relaxation.

4. **Yoga:** Yoga combines physical postures, breathing exercises, and meditation to promote relaxation and reduce stress. Regular yoga practice has been shown to lower cortisol levels, decrease anxiety, and improve overall well-being. Many yoga studios and online platforms offer classes for practitioners of all levels.

5. **Exercise:** Physical activity, such as walking, jogging, swimming, or dancing, can help reduce stress by releasing endorphins, which are natural mood lifters. To experience the benefits of stress relief, try to get in at least 30 minutes of moderate-intensity exercise most days of the week.

6. **Spending Time in Nature:** Spending time outdoors in nature can have a calming effect on the mind and body. Take a walk in the park, hike in the woods, or simply sit and enjoy the beauty of your surroundings. Reducing stress and enhancing general wellbeing can be achieved via connecting with nature.

7. **Journaling:** Writing down your thoughts and feelings in a journal can help you process emotions, gain perspective, and identify sources of stress. Try setting aside a few minutes each day to journal about your thoughts, experiences, and gratitude.

8. **Social Support:** Talking to friends, family members, or a therapist about your stressors can provide emotional support and perspective. Having a strong support network can help buffer the effects of stress and promote resilience.

9. **Healthy Lifestyle Habits:** Engaging in healthy lifestyle habits, such as eating a balanced diet, getting enough sleep, and limiting caffeine and alcohol intake, can help support overall well-being and reduce stress levels.

By incorporating these stress management techniques into your daily routine, you can better cope with stress, promote relaxation, and support your overall health, including gut health.

IMPORTANCE OF SLEEP

Sleep is crucial for overall health and well-being, playing a vital role in various physiological processes and bodily functions. Here are some key reasons highlighting the importance of sleep:

1. **Restoration and Repair:** During sleep, the body undergoes essential processes of restoration and repair. Tissues and muscles are repaired, and growth hormones are released to support growth and development, particularly in children and adolescents.

2. **Cognitive Function:** Adequate sleep is essential for optimal cognitive function, including memory consolidation, problem-solving abilities, decision-making skills, and concentration. Getting enough sleep improves learning and enhances overall cognitive performance.

3. **Emotional Regulation:** Sleep plays a crucial role in regulating emotions and mood. Chronic sleep deprivation can lead to irritability, mood swings, increased stress levels, and a higher risk of developing mood disorders such as depression and anxiety.

4. **Immune Function:** Sleep is vital for a healthy immune system. The body creates cytokines, which are proteins that aid in controlling the immune system's reaction to infections and inflammation, while you sleep. People who experience long-term sleep deprivation are more vulnerable to infections and illnesses because their immune systems are weakened.

5. **Metabolic Health:** Sleep plays a significant role in regulating metabolism and appetite. Lack of sleep can disrupt hormone levels, leading to increased hunger and cravings for high-calorie foods. Chronic sleep deprivation is associated with weight gain, obesity, insulin resistance, and an increased risk of type 2 diabetes.

6. **Cardiovascular Health:** Adequate sleep is crucial for maintaining cardiovascular health. Chronic sleep deprivation is linked to an increased risk of hypertension (high blood pressure), heart disease, stroke, and irregular heart rhythms.

7. **Mental Health:** Sleep and mental health are closely intertwined. Adequate sleep is essential for emotional well-being and resilience, while sleep disturbances can exacerbate symptoms of mental health disorders such as depression and anxiety.

8. **Overall Well-being:** Quality sleep is fundamental for overall physical, mental, and emotional well-being. It promotes feelings of vitality, energy, and vitality, allowing individuals to function optimally throughout the day.

In summary, sleep is a fundamental aspect of health and plays a critical role in numerous bodily functions and processes. Prioritizing sleep and adopting healthy sleep habits is essential for maintaining overall health, vitality, and quality of life.

EXERCISE AND GUT HEALTH

Exercise has numerous benefits for overall health, including its positive impact on gut health. Here's how exercise can contribute to a healthy gut:

1. **Promotes Gut Motility:** Regular physical activity can help stimulate bowel movements and promote regularity. Exercise helps to keep the muscles of the digestive tract strong and functioning efficiently, reducing the risk of constipation and promoting healthy bowel habits.

2. **Reduces Gut Inflammation:** Chronic inflammation in the gut is associated with various digestive disorders, including inflammatory bowel diseases (IBD) like Crohn's disease and ulcerative colitis. Exercise has anti-inflammatory effects on the body, which can help reduce inflammation in the gut and alleviate symptoms of digestive disorders.

3. **Modulates Gut Microbiota:** Exercise can positively influence the composition and diversity of the gut microbiota, the trillions of bacteria that reside in the digestive tract. Regular physical activity has been shown to increase the abundance of beneficial bacteria, such as Lactobacillus and

Bifidobacterium, while reducing the levels of harmful bacteria. This balance of gut bacteria is essential for maintaining gut health and overall well-being.

4. **Enhances Gut Barrier Function:** The lining of the intestines acts as a barrier, regulating the passage of nutrients and preventing harmful substances from entering the bloodstream. Exercise has been shown to improve gut barrier function, strengthening the intestinal barrier and reducing the risk of leaky gut syndrome, a condition characterized by increased intestinal permeability.

5. **Improves Digestive Symptoms:** Exercise can help alleviate digestive symptoms such as bloating, gas, and abdominal discomfort. Physical activity promotes better digestion and can help relieve symptoms of conditions like irritable bowel syndrome (IBS) by reducing stress and promoting relaxation.

6. **Supports Weight Management:** Regular exercise is essential for maintaining a healthy weight, which is crucial for gut health. Obesity and excess body fat are risk factors for various digestive disorders, including GERD (gastroesophageal reflux disease), gallstones, and fatty liver disease. By promoting weight loss and weight maintenance, exercise can help reduce the risk of these conditions and support overall gut health.

7. **Enhances Overall Well-being:** In addition to its direct effects on gut health, exercise has numerous indirect benefits for overall well-being, including reduced stress, improved mood, better sleep quality, and increased energy levels. These factors can all contribute to better digestive health and overall quality of life.

In conclusion, regular exercise is essential for promoting a healthy gut and overall digestive wellness. By incorporating physical activity into your daily routine, you can support optimal gut function, reduce the risk of digestive disorders, and improve your overall health and well-being.

CHAPTER SIX

SPECIAL CONSIDERATIONS FOR WOMEN'S HEALTH

Women's health encompasses a range of unique considerations, including reproductive health, hormonal fluctuations, and specific health conditions that affect women disproportionately. Here are some special considerations for women's health:

1. **Reproductive Health:** Women experience reproductive health milestones such as menstruation, pregnancy, childbirth, and menopause. Regular gynecological exams, including Pap smears and breast exams, are essential for early detection of conditions such as cervical cancer and breast cancer.

2. **Hormonal Fluctuations:** Hormonal changes throughout a woman's life, including during menstruation, pregnancy, and menopause, can affect various aspects of health, including mood, energy levels, metabolism, and bone health. Understanding and managing hormonal fluctuations are crucial for maintaining overall well-being.

3. **Birth Control and Family Planning:** Women have unique contraceptive needs, and choosing the

right birth control method is important for preventing unintended pregnancies and managing reproductive health. Family planning services, including access to contraception and preconception counseling, are essential for women's health.

4. **Menstrual Health:** Menstrual disorders such as irregular periods, heavy bleeding, and painful cramps are common among women. Addressing menstrual health concerns, including underlying conditions such as endometriosis or polycystic ovary syndrome (PCOS), is important for managing symptoms and promoting overall well-being.

5. **Bone Health:** Women are at higher risk of osteoporosis, a condition characterized by weakened bones and increased fracture risk, especially after menopause. Adequate calcium and vitamin D intake, weight-bearing exercise, and lifestyle modifications are important for maintaining bone health and reducing the risk of osteoporosis.

6. **Heart Health:** Heart disease is the leading cause of death among women worldwide. Women may experience different heart disease symptoms than men, and certain risk factors, such as pregnancy complications and hormonal birth control, can affect heart health. Understanding heart disease risk factors and adopting heart-healthy lifestyle habits are essential for preventing cardiovascular disease in women.

7. **Breast Health:** Breast cancer is the most common cancer among women globally. Regular breast self-exams, clinical breast exams, and mammograms are important for early detection and treatment of breast cancer. Breastfeeding and maintaining a healthy weight may also reduce the risk of breast cancer.

8. **Mental Health:** Women are more likely than men to experience mental health conditions such as depression and anxiety. Hormonal fluctuations, life transitions, and social factors can contribute to mental health challenges in women. Access to mental health services, support networks, and self-care strategies are essential for promoting mental well-being.

9. **Sexual and Reproductive Rights:** Ensuring women's access to comprehensive sexual and reproductive health care, including contraception, abortion services, and maternal health care, is essential for promoting women's health and autonomy.

10. **Gender-Specific Conditions:** Women may also experience gender-specific health conditions such as ovarian cancer, endometriosis, and pelvic floor disorders. Awareness, early detection, and appropriate management of these conditions are critical for maintaining women's health and quality of life.

By addressing these special considerations and prioritizing women's unique health needs, individuals, healthcare providers, and policymakers can work together to promote optimal health outcomes for women across the lifespan.

GUT HEALTH AND HORMONAL BALANCE

Gut health and hormonal balance are interconnected in various ways, as the gut and hormones influence each other through a complex network of interactions. Here are some key points highlighting the relationship between gut health and hormonal balance:

1. **Gut Microbiota and Hormonal Regulation:** The gut microbiota, comprised of trillions of bacteria, plays a crucial role in hormonal regulation. Certain gut bacteria are involved in the metabolism and synthesis of hormones, including estrogen, progesterone, and testosterone. Imbalances in the gut microbiota can disrupt hormonal signaling pathways, leading to hormonal imbalances.

2. **Estrogen Metabolism:** The gut microbiota plays a role in metabolizing estrogen and removing it from the body. Dysbiosis, or an imbalance in gut bacteria, can affect estrogen metabolism, leading to alterations in estrogen levels. This imbalance may

contribute to conditions such as estrogen dominance or estrogen deficiency.

3. **Gut Hormones:** The gut produces several hormones, including ghrelin, leptin, and peptide YY, which regulate appetite, metabolism, and energy balance. Imbalances in gut hormones can affect appetite regulation, leading to weight gain or obesity, which in turn can impact hormonal balance.

4. **Inflammation and Hormonal Imbalance:** Dysbiosis and intestinal permeability (leaky gut) can lead to chronic inflammation in the gut, which can disrupt hormonal balance. Inflammatory cytokines produced in the gut can interfere with the production, release, and function of hormones, contributing to hormonal imbalances.

5. **Stress and Gut Health:** Chronic stress can disrupt gut health by altering gut motility, increasing intestinal permeability, and affecting the composition of the gut microbiota. Stress hormones such as cortisol can impact gut function and exacerbate gastrointestinal symptoms. In turn, gut dysbiosis and inflammation resulting from stress can further disrupt hormonal balance.

6. **Thyroid Function:** The gut microbiota may influence thyroid hormone metabolism and function. Imbalances in gut bacteria, as well as gut inflammation, can affect thyroid hormone levels and thyroid function. Conditions such as Hashimoto's

thyroiditis, an autoimmune thyroid disorder, may be influenced by gut health and inflammation.

7. **Hormonal Birth Control:** The use of hormonal contraceptives, such as birth control pills, can affect gut health by altering the composition of the gut microbiota and increasing intestinal permeability. These changes may contribute to gastrointestinal symptoms such as bloating, gas, and changes in bowel habits.

8. **Hormonal Changes During Menstrual Cycle:** Hormonal fluctuations during the menstrual cycle can impact gut function and symptoms such as bloating, constipation, or diarrhea. Progesterone, in particular, can affect gut motility and may contribute to changes in bowel habits.

Overall, maintaining a healthy gut microbiota, managing stress, and adopting lifestyle habits that support gut health, such as eating a balanced diet, staying hydrated, and getting regular exercise, are important for promoting hormonal balance. Working with healthcare providers to address gut health issues and hormonal imbalances can help optimize overall health and well-being.

PREGNANCY AND GUT HEALTH

During pregnancy, gut health plays a crucial role in supporting the overall health and well-being of both the mother and the developing fetus. Here are several ways in which pregnancy can impact gut health, and vice versa:

1. **Changes in Gut Microbiota:** Pregnancy is associated with changes in the composition and diversity of the gut microbiota. These changes are thought to be influenced by hormonal fluctuations, immune system modulation, and dietary habits. Maintaining a healthy balance of gut bacteria during pregnancy is important for supporting maternal health and potentially influencing the long-term health of the offspring.

2. **Digestive Symptoms:** Pregnant women often experience digestive symptoms such as nausea, vomiting, constipation, and heartburn due to hormonal changes, increased progesterone levels, and pressure from the growing uterus on the digestive organs. These symptoms can impact gut health and may require dietary and lifestyle modifications to manage effectively.

3. **Nutrient Absorption:** Adequate nutrient absorption is essential during pregnancy to support fetal growth and development. Gut health plays a critical role in nutrient absorption, and conditions such as gastrointestinal disorders or malabsorption

syndromes can affect nutrient uptake. Ensuring optimal gut health through a balanced diet and prenatal supplements can support nutrient absorption during pregnancy.

4. **Immune Function:** The gut plays a central role in immune function, and maintaining a healthy gut microbiota is important for supporting maternal immune health during pregnancy. A balanced gut microbiota can help prevent infections and reduce the risk of complications such as preterm birth or preeclampsia.

5. **Gestational Diabetes:** Gestational diabetes is a condition characterized by high blood sugar levels during pregnancy. Recent research suggests that alterations in gut microbiota composition and function may contribute to the development of gestational diabetes. Modifying dietary habits and lifestyle factors to support gut health may help reduce the risk of gestational diabetes.

6. **Gut-Brain Axis:** The gut-brain axis, which involves bidirectional communication between the gut and the brain, plays a role in regulating mood, stress responses, and mental health. Pregnancy-related stress and changes in gut microbiota composition may impact the gut-brain axis, potentially influencing maternal mental health and well-being during pregnancy.

7. **Postpartum Recovery:** After childbirth, the gut microbiota undergoes further changes as the body transitions to the postpartum period. Breastfeeding can also influence maternal gut health, as breast milk contains nutrients and bioactive compounds that support the growth of beneficial gut bacteria in both the mother and the infant.

Overall, maintaining a healthy gut microbiota through a balanced diet, probiotic supplementation (under the guidance of a healthcare provider), regular physical activity, and stress management techniques is important for supporting maternal health and promoting optimal outcomes during pregnancy. Consulting with a healthcare provider for personalized recommendations can help address any specific gut health concerns during pregnancy.

MENOPAUSE AND GUT HEALTH

Menopause is a natural transition in a woman's life marked by the cessation of menstruation and a decline in reproductive hormone levels, particularly estrogen and progesterone. This hormonal shift can have various effects on the body, including changes in gut health. Here's how menopause can impact gut health:

1. **Changes in Gut Microbiota:** Menopause is associated with alterations in the composition and diversity of the gut microbiota. Estrogen and progesterone influence the gut microbiota composition, and their decline during menopause can lead to shifts in the abundance of certain bacteria. These changes may affect gut function, nutrient absorption, and metabolism.

2. **Digestive Symptoms:** Menopausal women may experience digestive symptoms such as bloating, gas, constipation, or diarrhea. These symptoms can be attributed to hormonal fluctuations, changes in gut motility, alterations in gut microbiota, and lifestyle factors. Managing digestive symptoms through dietary modifications, probiotics, and lifestyle changes can help support gut health during menopause.

3. **Weight Gain and Metabolism:** Many women experience weight gain, particularly around the abdomen, during menopause. This may be related to hormonal changes, decreased physical activity, and changes in metabolism. Excess weight and central obesity are associated with an increased risk of metabolic disorders and cardiovascular disease, which can impact gut health and overall well-being.

4. **Bone Health:** Estrogen plays a crucial role in maintaining bone health, and its decline during menopause can lead to bone loss and an increased

risk of osteoporosis. Gut health is closely linked to bone health, as the gut microbiota can influence calcium absorption and bone metabolism. Supporting gut health through a balanced diet and probiotics may help optimize bone health during menopause.

5. **Hormonal Therapy:** Hormone replacement therapy (HRT) is commonly used to alleviate menopausal symptoms by replacing estrogen and/or progesterone. HRT may have implications for gut health, as estrogen and progesterone influence gut microbiota composition and function. Further research is needed to understand the effects of HRT on gut health and whether it impacts gastrointestinal symptoms or disorders.

6. **Mental Health:** Menopause is associated with an increased risk of mood disturbances, anxiety, and depression. Gut health and mental health are interconnected through the gut-brain axis, which involves bidirectional communication between the gut and the brain. Supporting gut health through dietary interventions and probiotics may have beneficial effects on mood and mental well-being during menopause.

7. **Cardiovascular Health:** Estrogen has cardioprotective effects, and its decline during menopause is associated with an increased risk of cardiovascular disease. Maintaining gut health is important for cardiovascular health, as gut microbiota composition and function can influence cardiovascular risk factors such as inflammation, lipid metabolism, and blood pressure.

Overall, supporting gut health through dietary interventions, probiotics, regular physical activity, and stress management techniques can help mitigate menopause-related symptoms and promote overall well-being during this transitional phase of life. Consulting with a healthcare provider for personalized recommendations and management strategies is important for addressing menopause-related gut health concerns.

CHAPTER SEVEN

SUPPLEMENTS FOR GUT HEALTH

Supplements can be a helpful addition to support gut health, especially when combined with a healthy diet and lifestyle. Here are some supplements commonly used to promote gut health:

1. **Probiotics:** Probiotics are live beneficial bacteria that can help restore and maintain a healthy balance of gut microbiota. They may help alleviate digestive symptoms such as bloating, gas, and diarrhea, and support immune function. Look for probiotic supplements containing a variety of strains, including Lactobacillus and Bifidobacterium species.

2. **Prebiotics:** Prebiotics are non-digestible fibers that serve as food for beneficial gut bacteria, helping them thrive and multiply. They can be found naturally in foods like onions, garlic, bananas, and asparagus, or taken as supplements. Incorporating prebiotic supplements or foods into your diet can help support the growth of beneficial gut bacteria.

3. **Fiber Supplements:** Fiber is essential for maintaining regular bowel movements and

supporting overall gut health. If you're not getting enough fiber from your diet, fiber supplements such as psyllium husk, glucomannan, or acacia fiber can help promote bowel regularity and support digestive health.

4. **Digestive Enzymes:** Digestive enzymes help break down carbohydrates, proteins, and fats in the digestive tract, aiding in nutrient absorption and reducing digestive discomfort. Supplementing with digestive enzymes may be beneficial for individuals with conditions such as pancreatic insufficiency or irritable bowel syndrome (IBS).

5. **L-Glutamine:** L-Glutamine is an amino acid that plays a crucial role in maintaining the integrity of the intestinal lining and supporting gut barrier function. It may help alleviate symptoms of leaky gut syndrome and promote gut healing. L-Glutamine supplements are available in powder or capsule form.

6. **Fish Oil/Omega-3 Fatty Acids:** Omega-3 fatty acids have anti-inflammatory properties and may help reduce inflammation in the gut. Fish oil supplements, rich in EPA and DHA, can support gut health and may be beneficial for individuals with inflammatory bowel diseases (IBD) or other inflammatory conditions.

7. **Collagen:** Collagen is a protein that provides structural support to the intestinal lining and helps

maintain gut integrity. Supplementing with collagen peptides may support gut health and promote healing of the gut lining, especially in individuals with conditions such as leaky gut syndrome or irritable bowel syndrome (IBS).

8. **Herbal Supplements:** Certain herbs and botanicals have been traditionally used to support digestive health. Examples include licorice root, slippery elm bark, marshmallow root, and ginger. These herbs may help soothe digestive discomfort and promote gastrointestinal wellness.

It's essential to consult with a healthcare provider before starting any new supplement regimen, especially if you have pre-existing health conditions or are taking medications. Additionally, aim to obtain nutrients from a varied and balanced diet whenever possible, as supplements should complement, not replace, a healthy lifestyle.

UNDERSTANDING SUPPLEMENTS OPTIONS

Understanding supplement options involves knowing the types of supplements available, their intended purposes, and potential benefits. Here's an overview of common supplement categories:

1. **Vitamins:** Vitamins are essential micronutrients that the body needs for various

functions, including metabolism, immune function, and tissue repair. Common vitamins include vitamin A, vitamin C, vitamin D, vitamin E, and the B vitamins (B1, B2, B3, B5, B6, B7, B9, B12). Vitamin supplements are often used to fill nutrient gaps in the diet or to address specific deficiencies.

2. **Minerals:** Minerals are inorganic compounds that play vital roles in bodily functions, such as bone health, nerve function, and muscle contraction. Common minerals include calcium, magnesium, iron, zinc, selenium, and potassium. Mineral supplements may be used to support overall health or to address specific deficiencies.

3. **Probiotics:** Probiotics are live beneficial bacteria that support gut health and digestion. They can help restore the balance of gut microbiota, alleviate digestive symptoms, and support immune function. Probiotic supplements typically contain strains of Lactobacillus and Bifidobacterium bacteria.

4. **Prebiotics:** Prebiotics are non-digestible fibers that serve as food for beneficial gut bacteria. They help promote the growth of probiotic bacteria in the gut and support overall gut health. Prebiotic supplements may contain fibers such as inulin, fructooligosaccharides (FOS), or galactooligosaccharides (GOS).

5. **Omega-3 Fatty Acids:** Omega-3 fatty acids are essential fats that are important for heart health, brain function, and inflammation regulation. They are found in fatty fish, flaxseeds, chia seeds, and walnuts. Omega-3 supplements typically contain EPA (eicosapentaenoic acid) and DHA (docosahexaenoic acid) derived from fish oil or algae.

6. **Herbal Supplements:** Herbal supplements are derived from plants and may be used for various purposes, including supporting overall health, promoting relaxation, boosting immunity, or addressing specific health concerns. Examples of herbal supplements include echinacea, turmeric, ginger, and ginseng.

7. **Amino Acids:** Amino acids are the building blocks of proteins and are essential for various bodily functions, including muscle repair, neurotransmitter synthesis, and hormone production. Some amino acids, such as glutamine and branched-chain amino acids (BCAAs), are available as supplements and may be used to support muscle recovery, gut health, or athletic performance.

8. **Joint Health Supplements:** Joint health supplements may contain ingredients such as glucosamine, chondroitin, MSM (methylsulfonylmethane), and collagen peptides. These supplements are commonly used to support

joint health, reduce inflammation, and alleviate symptoms of conditions such as osteoarthritis.

Before starting any new supplement regimen, it's essential to consult with a healthcare provider, especially if you have pre-existing health conditions, are pregnant or breastfeeding, or are taking medications. Additionally, aim to obtain nutrients from a varied and balanced diet whenever possible, as supplements should complement, not replace, a healthy lifestyle.

RECOMMENDED SUPPLEMENTS FOR WOMEN

Recommended supplements for women can vary depending on individual health needs, dietary habits, lifestyle factors, and life stages. However, some supplements are commonly recommended for women to support overall health and well-being. Here are several supplements that may be beneficial for women:

1. **Multivitamin:** A high-quality multivitamin can help fill nutrient gaps in the diet and provide essential vitamins and minerals that may be lacking. Look for a multivitamin specifically formulated for women that contains adequate amounts of key nutrients such as vitamin D, calcium, iron, magnesium, and B vitamins.

2. **Calcium:** Women are at a higher risk of osteoporosis, a condition characterized by weakened bones, especially after menopause. Calcium supplements can help support bone health and reduce the risk of fractures. Look for calcium supplements that also contain vitamin D and magnesium, which aid in calcium absorption.

3. **Vitamin D:** Vitamin D is essential for bone health, immune function, and mood regulation. Many people, including women, have insufficient vitamin D levels, especially those who live in northern latitudes or have limited sun exposure. Vitamin D supplements can help maintain optimal vitamin D levels.

4. **Omega-3 Fatty Acids:** Omega-3 fatty acids, particularly EPA and DHA, are important for heart health, brain function, and inflammation regulation. Omega-3 supplements derived from fish oil or algae can help support cardiovascular health and cognitive function.

5. **Iron:** Iron is essential for the production of red blood cells and oxygen transport in the body. Women of childbearing age, especially those who menstruate heavily, are at risk of iron deficiency anemia. Iron supplements may be recommended for women with iron deficiency or those at risk of deficiency.

6. **Probiotics:** Probiotics are beneficial bacteria that support gut health and digestion. They may help alleviate digestive symptoms such as bloating, gas, and constipation, and support immune function. Look for probiotic supplements containing a variety of strains, including Lactobacillus and Bifidobacterium species.

7. **Folic Acid (Folate):** Folic acid is essential for fetal development during pregnancy and helps prevent neural tube defects in newborns. Women of childbearing age, especially those planning to become pregnant, should ensure adequate intake of folic acid through diet and/or supplements.

8. **Magnesium:** Magnesium is involved in over 300 biochemical reactions in the body and plays a role in muscle function, energy metabolism, and bone health. Many women have inadequate magnesium intake, and supplements may be beneficial for those with low magnesium levels or deficiency.

9. **Collagen:** Collagen is a protein that provides structural support to the skin, joints, and bones. Collagen supplements may help improve skin elasticity, joint health, and bone density in women, especially as they age.

Before starting any new supplement regimen, it's important to consult with a healthcare provider, especially if you have pre-existing health conditions, are pregnant or breastfeeding, or are taking medications. Additionally, aim to obtain nutrients from a varied and balanced diet whenever possible, as supplements should complement, not replace, a healthy lifestyle.

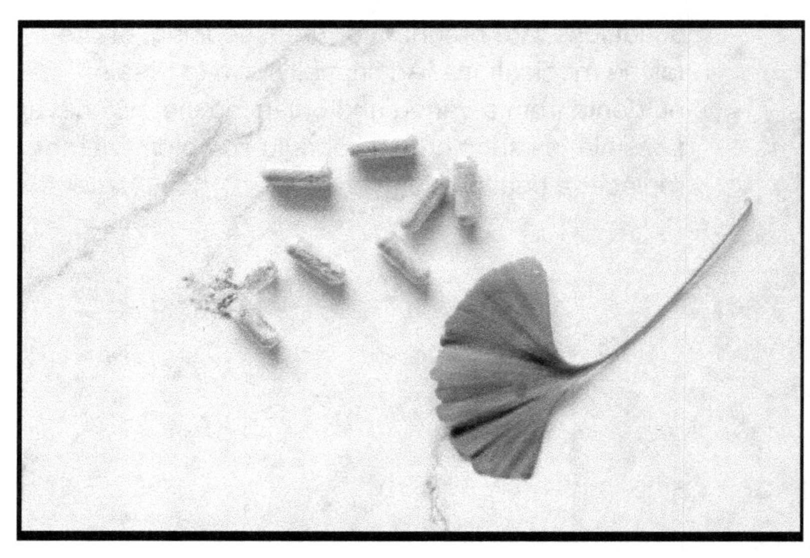

CHAPTER EIGHT

TROUBLESHOOTING COMMON GUT ISSUES

Troubleshooting common gut issues involves identifying the underlying causes and implementing strategies to alleviate symptoms and promote gut health. Here are some common gut issues and strategies for troubleshooting them:

1. **Bloating and Gas:**
- **Identify trigger foods:** Certain foods, such as beans, cruciferous vegetables, dairy products, and artificial sweeteners, can cause bloating and gas in some individuals. Keep a food diary to track symptoms and identify potential triggers.
- **Eat smaller meals:** Large meals can put additional strain on the digestive system and exacerbate bloating and gas. Eat smaller, more frequent meals throughout the day to support digestion.
- **Chew food thoroughly:** Properly chewing food can aid digestion and reduce the likelihood of swallowing air, which can contribute to bloating and gas.
- **Consider probiotics:** Probiotic supplements or probiotic-rich foods like yogurt, kefir, and sauerkraut may help restore balance to the gut microbiota and alleviate bloating and gas.

2. **Constipation:**
   - **Increase fiber intake:** Fiber helps promote bowel regularity by adding bulk to stool and supporting healthy digestion. Incorporate fiber-rich foods such as fruits, vegetables, whole grains, legumes, and nuts into your diet.
   - **Stay hydrated:** Drinking plenty of water throughout the day can help soften stool and facilitate bowel movements. Aim for at least eight glasses of water per day, and limit dehydrating beverages like caffeine and alcohol.
   - **Get regular exercise:** Physical activity helps stimulate bowel movements and promote gut motility. On most days of the week, try to get in at least 30 minutes of moderate-intensity exercise.
   - **Consider fiber supplements:** If dietary changes alone are not sufficient, fiber supplements such as psyllium husk or methylcellulose may help alleviate constipation.

3. **Diarrhea:**
   - **Identify trigger foods:** Certain foods and beverages, such as spicy foods, fatty foods, caffeine, and alcohol, can exacerbate diarrhea in some individuals. Avoiding trigger foods may help alleviate symptoms.
   - **Stay hydrated:** Diarrhea can lead to dehydration, so it's essential to drink plenty of fluids to replenish lost electrolytes and maintain hydration.

- **Consider probiotics:** Probiotic supplements or probiotic-rich foods may help restore balance to the gut microbiota and alleviate diarrhea, especially if it is caused by antibiotic use or infection.
- **Practice good hygiene:** Wash hands frequently, especially before eating and after using the restroom, to prevent the spread of infectious diarrhea.

4. **Heartburn and Acid Reflux:**

- **Avoid trigger foods:** Certain foods and beverages, such as spicy foods, citrus fruits, tomatoes, coffee, and alcohol, can trigger heartburn and acid reflux. Identify and avoid your personal trigger foods.
- **Eat smaller meals:** Large meals can increase pressure on the lower esophageal sphincter (LES) and contribute to acid reflux. Opt for smaller, more frequent meals to reduce the risk of heartburn.
- **Avoid lying down after eating:** Wait at least two to three hours after eating before lying down or going to bed to allow time for digestion and reduce the likelihood of acid reflux.
- **Elevate the head of the bed:** Sleeping with the head of the bed elevated may help prevent acid reflux by keeping stomach acid from flowing back into the esophagus.

5. **Leaky Gut Syndrome:**

- **Address underlying causes:** Leaky gut syndrome may be caused by factors such as chronic stress, poor diet, medications, infections, or underlying health conditions. Identify and address the underlying causes to promote gut healing.

- **Follow a gut-healing diet:** Eliminate inflammatory foods such as processed foods, refined sugars, gluten, and dairy, and focus on whole, nutrient-dense foods that support gut health, such as fruits, vegetables, lean proteins, and healthy fats.

- **Support gut healing:** Incorporate supplements such as L-glutamine, collagen, zinc, and digestive enzymes to support gut healing and repair the intestinal lining.

- **Manage stress:** Chronic stress can contribute to leaky gut syndrome by disrupting gut barrier function. Practice stress management techniques such as mindfulness meditation, deep breathing exercises, yoga, or regular exercise to reduce stress levels and support gut health.

It's important to note that persistent or severe gut issues should be evaluated by a healthcare professional to rule out underlying medical conditions and determine the most appropriate course of treatment. Additionally, individual responses to dietary and lifestyle changes may vary, so it may be helpful to work with a registered dietitian or healthcare provider to develop a personalized plan for troubleshooting gut issues.

BLOATING AND DIGESTIVE DISCOMFORT

Bloating and digestive discomfort are common complaints that can be caused by various factors, including diet, lifestyle, and underlying digestive issues. Here are some strategies to help alleviate bloating and digestive discomfort:

1. **Identify Trigger Foods:** Keep a food diary to track your symptoms and identify any foods that may be causing bloating or discomfort. Common trigger foods include beans, cruciferous vegetables (such as broccoli and cabbage), dairy products, gluten-containing grains, artificial sweeteners, and carbonated beverages. Once identified, try eliminating or reducing these foods from your diet to see if your symptoms improve.

2. **Eat Mindfully:** Chew your food slowly and thoroughly, and avoid swallowing air while eating, as this can contribute to bloating. Eating too quickly or gulping down food and beverages can introduce excess air into the digestive tract, leading to gas and bloating. Try to relax and enjoy your meals in a calm environment.

3. **Limit Gas-Producing Foods:** Some foods are known to produce gas in the digestive tract, leading to bloating and discomfort. These include beans, lentils, onions, garlic, Brussels sprouts, cauliflower, and certain fruits (such as apples,

pears, and stone fruits). While these foods are nutritious, you may want to limit your intake or choose alternative cooking methods (such as soaking beans before cooking) to reduce gas production.

4. **Manage Stress:** Chronic stress can affect digestion and contribute to bloating and digestive discomfort. Engage in stress-relieving activities like yoga, meditation, deep breathing, and spending time in nature. Finding ways to relax and unwind can help improve overall digestive health.

5. **Stay Hydrated:** Drink plenty of water throughout the day to support healthy digestion and prevent constipation, which can contribute to bloating. Aim for at least eight glasses of water per day, and limit caffeine and alcohol, which can dehydrate the body and exacerbate digestive issues.

6. **Probiotics:** Consider incorporating probiotic-rich foods (such as yogurt, kefir, sauerkraut, and kimchi) into your diet or taking a probiotic supplement. Probiotics can help restore balance to the gut microbiota and alleviate symptoms of bloating and digestive discomfort in some individuals.

7. **Fiber Intake:** Gradually increase your intake of soluble fiber-rich foods, such as oats, bananas, apples, and legumes, which can help regulate

bowel movements and alleviate constipation. However, be mindful not to increase fiber intake too quickly, as this can exacerbate bloating and gas in some people. Drink plenty of water when increasing fiber intake to help prevent digestive discomfort.

8. **Seek Medical Advice:** If bloating and digestive discomfort persist despite dietary and lifestyle modifications, or if you experience other concerning symptoms such as abdominal pain, changes in bowel habits, or unintended weight loss, consult with a healthcare professional. They can help identify any underlying digestive issues and recommend appropriate treatment options.

By implementing these strategies and making gradual changes to your diet and lifestyle, you can help alleviate bloating and digestive discomfort and promote overall digestive health.

CONSTIPATION AND DIARRHEA

Constipation and diarrhea are common digestive issues that can be caused by various factors, including diet, lifestyle, medications, and underlying health conditions. Here are some strategies to help alleviate constipation and diarrhea:

Constipation:

1. **Increase Fiber Intake:** Eat a diet rich in fiber from fruits, vegetables, whole grains, legumes, and nuts. Fiber gives stools more volume and encourages regular bowel motions. Aim for 25–30 grams of fiber each day to maintain the healthiest possible gut.

2. **Stay Hydrated:** Drink plenty of water throughout the day to help soften stool and facilitate bowel movements. Aim for at least eight glasses of water per day, and limit dehydrating beverages such as caffeine and alcohol.

3. **Regular Exercise:** Engage in regular physical activity to stimulate bowel movements and promote gut motility. On most days of the week, try to get in at least 30 minutes of moderate-intensity exercise.

4. **Establish a Routine:** Try to establish a regular bowel movement routine by going to the bathroom at the same time each day, preferably after meals or in the morning when bowel movements are most likely to happen.

5. **Consider Fiber Supplements:** If increasing dietary fiber alone is not sufficient, consider taking a fiber supplement such as psyllium husk or methylcellulose. These supplements can help add bulk to stool and promote regular bowel movements.

6. **Probiotics:** Probiotic supplements or probiotic-rich foods like yogurt, kefir, and sauerkraut may help restore balance to the gut microbiota and alleviate constipation in some individuals.

7. **Limit Processed Foods:** Processed foods that are low in fiber and high in refined sugars and fats can contribute to constipation. Opt for whole, nutrient-dense foods whenever possible, and limit processed and refined foods.

8. **Manage Stress:** Chronic stress can affect gut motility and contribute to constipation. Practice stress management techniques such as mindfulness meditation, deep breathing exercises, or yoga to reduce stress levels and support digestive health.

Diarrhea:

1. **Stay Hydrated:** Drink plenty of fluids to prevent dehydration and replenish lost electrolytes. Clear liquids such as water, broth, and electrolyte drinks are especially important during episodes of diarrhea.

2. **BRAT Diet:** Follow a bland diet consisting of bananas, rice, applesauce, and toast (BRAT) to help firm up stool and alleviate diarrhea. These foods are easy to digest and can help settle the stomach.

3. **Avoid Trigger Foods:** Identify and avoid foods and beverages that may trigger diarrhea, such as spicy foods, fatty foods, dairy products (if lactose intolerant), caffeine, and artificial sweeteners.

4. **Probiotics:** Probiotic supplements or probiotic-rich foods may help restore balance to the gut microbiota and alleviate diarrhea, especially if it is caused by antibiotic use or infection.

5. **BRAT Diet:** Follow a bland diet consisting of bananas, rice, applesauce, and toast (BRAT) to help firm up stool and alleviate diarrhea. These foods are easy to digest and can help settle the stomach.

6. **Avoid Trigger Foods:** Identify and avoid foods and beverages that may trigger diarrhea, such as spicy foods, fatty foods, dairy products (if lactose intolerant), caffeine, and artificial sweeteners.

7. **Probiotics:** Probiotic supplements or probiotic-rich foods may help restore balance to the gut microbiota and alleviate diarrhea, especially if it is caused by antibiotic use or infection.

8. **Over-the-Counter Medications:**
Over-the-counter anti-diarrheal medications such as loperamide (Imodium) or bismuth subsalicylate (Pepto-Bismol) may help alleviate symptoms of

acute diarrhea. However, it's important to use these medications as directed and consult with a healthcare professional if diarrhea persists or worsens.

9. **Seek Medical Advice:** If diarrhea is severe, persistent, or accompanied by other concerning symptoms such as fever, abdominal pain, or bloody stool, seek medical advice promptly. Chronic diarrhea may be a sign of underlying digestive issues that require medical evaluation and treatment.

By implementing these strategies and making dietary and lifestyle changes, you can help alleviate symptoms of constipation and diarrhea and promote overall digestive health. If symptoms persist or worsen, consult with a healthcare professional for further evaluation and personalized treatment recommendations.

MANAGING FOOD SENSITIVITIES AND ALLERGIES

Managing food sensitivities and allergies involves identifying trigger foods, avoiding exposure to allergens, and implementing strategies to prevent adverse reactions. Here are some tips for managing food sensitivities and allergies:

Food Sensitivities:

1. **Keep a Food Diary:** Keep a detailed record of the foods you eat and any symptoms you experience afterward. This can help identify patterns and potential trigger foods.

2. **Elimination Diet:** Consider doing an elimination diet to identify food sensitivities. Start by eliminating common trigger foods such as dairy, gluten, soy, eggs, and nuts for a few weeks, then gradually reintroduce them one at a time while monitoring for symptoms.

3. **Read Food Labels:** Pay close attention to food labels and ingredient lists to identify potential allergens and hidden sources of trigger foods.

4. **Cook at Home:** Cook meals at home with fresh, whole ingredients whenever possible. This gives you better control over the ingredients and reduces the risk of exposure to trigger foods.

5. **Consult with a Dietitian:** Consider working with a registered dietitian or nutritionist who specializes in food sensitivities. They can assist you in creating a personalized nutrition plan as well as providing advice on recognizing and controlling trigger foods.

6. **Consider Food Sensitivity Testing:** Talk to your healthcare provider about food sensitivity testing, such as IgG or IgE blood tests. While these

tests are not always definitive, they can provide useful information to guide an elimination diet.

Food Allergies:

1. **Know Your Triggers:** Identify and avoid foods that trigger allergic reactions. Common food allergens include peanuts, tree nuts, shellfish, fish, eggs, dairy, soy, and wheat.

2. **Read Labels Carefully:** Always read food labels carefully to identify potential allergens and cross-contamination risks. Manufacturers are required to label major food allergens, but cross-contamination can still occur.

3. **Communicate with Restaurants and Food Service Providers:** When dining out, inform restaurant staff about your food allergies and ask about ingredient lists and preparation methods. Choose restaurants that are knowledgeable about food allergies and take precautions to prevent cross-contamination.

4. **Carry Medication:** If you have a severe food allergy, such as to peanuts or shellfish, carry emergency medication such as an epinephrine auto-injector (e.g., EpiPen) with you at all times. Make sure your family members, friends, and coworkers know how to use it in case of an emergency.

5. **Create a Food Allergy Action Plan:** Work with your healthcare provider to create a personalized food allergy action plan that outlines steps to take in case of an allergic reaction. Share this plan with family members, caregivers, and others who may need to assist you in an emergency.

6. **Wear Medical Alert Identification:** Consider wearing a medical alert bracelet or necklace that indicates your food allergies. This can alert others to your condition in case of an emergency.

7. **Educate Others:** Educate family members, friends, coworkers, and caregivers about your food allergies and how to recognize and respond to an allergic reaction. Encourage them to be vigilant about reading food labels and taking precautions when preparing or serving food.

By taking proactive steps to identify trigger foods, avoid allergens, and communicate effectively with others, you can effectively manage food sensitivities and allergies and reduce the risk of adverse reactions. If you suspect you have a food allergy or sensitivity, consult with a healthcare professional for proper diagnosis and management.

CHAPTER NINE

MAINTAINING LONG-TERM GUT HEALTH

Maintaining long-term gut health involves adopting healthy habits that support the balance of gut microbiota, promote digestive function, and reduce the risk of gastrointestinal issues. Here are some strategies to help you maintain long-term gut health:

1. Eat a Diverse and Balanced Diet:
   - Consume a wide variety of fruits, vegetables, whole grains, lean proteins, and healthy fats to provide essential nutrients and support a diverse gut microbiota.
   - Include fiber-rich foods such as fruits, vegetables, legumes, and whole grains to promote bowel regularity and support digestive health.

2. Prioritize Gut-Friendly Foods:
   - Incorporate probiotic-rich foods such as yogurt, kefir, sauerkraut, kimchi, and miso into your diet to introduce beneficial bacteria to the gut.
   - Include prebiotic foods such as onions, garlic, leeks, bananas, asparagus, and whole grains to feed and nourish beneficial gut bacteria.

3. Stay Hydrated:

- Drink plenty of water throughout the day to support digestion, maintain bowel regularity, and prevent dehydration. Aim for at least 8-10 glasses of water per day.

4. Manage Stress:

- Practice stress-reducing techniques such as deep breathing, meditation, yoga, or mindfulness to help manage stress levels and promote gut health.
- Engage in regular physical activity, which can help reduce stress and support overall well-being.

5. Get Adequate Sleep:

- Aim for 7-9 hours of quality sleep per night to support overall health, including gut health. Poor sleep quality and inadequate sleep duration have been linked to disruptions in gut microbiota and digestive function.

6. Limit Processed Foods and Added Sugars:

- Minimize consumption of processed foods, sugary snacks, and sugary beverages, as these can disrupt gut microbiota balance and contribute to inflammation and digestive issues.

7. Limit Alcohol and Caffeine:

- Consume alcohol and caffeine in moderation, as excessive intake can irritate the gastrointestinal tract and disrupt gut health. Opt for water, herbal teas, or other non-alcoholic and caffeine-free beverages as alternatives.

8. Practice Good Food Hygiene:
   - Wash fruits and vegetables thoroughly before consuming them to remove dirt, bacteria, and pesticide residues.
   - Cook foods to the recommended temperature to kill harmful bacteria and reduce the risk of foodborne illnesses.

9. Avoid Smoking:
   - If you smoke, consider quitting smoking, as tobacco smoke can harm the digestive system and disrupt gut microbiota balance.

10. Regular Medical Check-Ups:
   - Schedule regular check-ups with your healthcare provider to monitor your overall health and address any gastrointestinal issues or concerns promptly.

By incorporating these habits into your daily routine, you can promote long-term gut health and support overall well-being. Remember that consistency is key, and small changes over time can lead to significant improvements in gut health and overall health. If you have specific concerns about your gut health or digestive function, consult with a healthcare professional for personalized advice and guidance.

STRATEGIES FOR SUSTAINABLE LIFESTYLE CHANGES

Making sustainable lifestyle changes involves adopting habits and behaviors that are realistic, enjoyable, and conducive to long-term success. Here are some strategies to help you make sustainable lifestyle changes:

1. Set Realistic Goals:
   - Set achievable goals that are specific, measurable, attainable, relevant, and time-bound (SMART). Break larger goals into smaller, more manageable steps to make progress gradually.

2. Focus on Behavior Change:
   - Instead of solely focusing on outcomes such as weight loss or improved fitness, focus on changing behaviors and habits that support your goals. For example, prioritize eating more vegetables, drinking more water, or exercising regularly.

3. Start Small:
   - Begin with small, manageable changes that you can easily incorporate into your daily routine. Once these changes become habits, gradually add more challenging goals or behaviors.

4. Be Flexible:
   - Be open to adjusting your goals and strategies as needed based on your progress, preferences, and circumstances. Life can be unpredictable, so

it's essential to adapt and find solutions that work for you.

5. Find Enjoyable Activities:
   - Choose physical activities and exercises that you enjoy and look forward to doing. Whether it's dancing, hiking, swimming, or playing sports, finding activities you enjoy makes it easier to stay active and motivated.

6. Make Healthier Food Choices:
   - Focus on adding more whole, nutrient-dense foods to your diet, such as fruits, vegetables, whole grains, lean proteins, and healthy fats. Aim for balance, variety, and moderation rather than strict rules or deprivation.

7. Practice Mindful Eating:
   - Pay attention to your body's hunger and fullness cues, and eat slowly and mindfully without distractions. Avoid emotional eating and practice self-awareness to make conscious food choices.

8. Get Support:
   - Surround yourself with supportive friends, family members, or peers who encourage and motivate you to make healthy choices. Consider joining a fitness class, support group, or online community for accountability and camaraderie.

9. Plan Ahead:

- Plan and prepare meals and snacks in advance to avoid impulsive or unhealthy food choices. Set aside time for meal planning, grocery shopping, and food prep each week to make healthy eating more convenient and accessible.

10. Practice Self-Compassion:

- Be kind to yourself and acknowledge that setbacks and challenges are a normal part of the process. Instead of dwelling on mistakes or perceived failures, focus on what you've learned and how you can move forward positively.

11. Celebrate Progress:

- No matter how minor, acknowledge and celebrate your victories and life milestones. Recognize your progress and reward yourself with non-food rewards such as a relaxing bath, a new workout outfit, or a fun activity you enjoy.

12. Stay Consistent:

- Consistency is key to making sustainable lifestyle changes. Stick to your new habits and routines even when motivation wanes or obstacles arise. Remember that every positive choice you make contributes to your overall progress and well-being.

By implementing these strategies and cultivating a positive mindset, you can make sustainable lifestyle changes that support your health, happiness, and long-term well-being. Remember that change takes time, patience, and persistence, so be kind to yourself as you work towards your goals.

TRACKING PROGRESS AND ADJUSTING GOALS

Tracking progress and adjusting goals are essential components of any successful lifestyle change journey. Here are some strategies to help you effectively track your progress and make adjustments to your goals:

1. Keep a Journal or Log:
   - Maintain a journal or log to track your daily habits, behaviors, and progress towards your goals. Record your food intake, exercise sessions, mood, energy levels, and any other relevant information that can help you evaluate your progress.

2. Use Technology:
   - Utilize technology tools such as mobile apps, fitness trackers, or online platforms to track your physical activity, nutrition, sleep, and other health-related metrics. These tools can provide valuable insights and help you stay accountable.

3. Measure Key Metrics:
   - Identify key metrics or indicators related to your goals and track them regularly. This could include body weight, body measurements, fitness levels,

blood pressure, cholesterol levels, or other health markers that are relevant to your objectives.

4. Set Milestones:

- Break your long-term goals into smaller milestones or checkpoints that you can aim to achieve along the way. Celebrate each milestone as you reach it, and use them as opportunities to assess your progress and adjust your approach if necessary.

5. Reflect Regularly:

- Take time to reflect on your progress, successes, and challenges regularly. Ask yourself what's working well, what could be improved, and what changes you need to make to stay on track towards your goals.

6. Be Honest with Yourself:

- Be honest and objective when evaluating your progress and adherence to your goals. Recognize areas where you may be falling short or struggling, and identify potential barriers or obstacles that may be hindering your progress.

7. Celebrate Achievements:

- Celebrate your achievements, no matter how small, and acknowledge the progress you've made towards your goals. Celebrating successes can boost motivation and reinforce positive behaviors.

8. Adjust Goals as Needed:

- Be flexible and willing to adjust your goals based on your progress, preferences, and changing circumstances. If you find that your original goals are no longer realistic or relevant, modify them accordingly to better align with your current needs and priorities.

9. Seek Feedback and Support:
   - Reach out to trusted friends, family members, or professionals for feedback and support. Share your progress, challenges, and goals with others who can offer encouragement, advice, and perspective.

10. Focus on Continuous Improvement:
   - Adopt an attitude that emphasizes lifelong learning and constant development. View setbacks and challenges as opportunities for growth and learning, and use them as motivation to keep moving forward towards your goals.

11. Stay Patient and Persistent:
   - Remember that progress takes time, and change doesn't happen overnight. Stay patient, stay persistent, and trust in the process as you work towards your goals. Stay committed to your journey, and don't be discouraged by temporary setbacks or obstacles.

By implementing these strategies and regularly monitoring your progress, you can effectively track your journey towards your goals and make adjustments as needed to ensure long-term success. Remember that personal growth and self-improvement are ongoing processes, and each step you take towards your goals is a step in the right direction.

CELEBRATING SUCCESS AND STAYING MOTIVATED

Celebrating success and staying motivated are crucial for maintaining momentum and achieving long-term goals. Here are some strategies to help you celebrate your successes and stay motivated throughout your journey:

1. Acknowledge Your Achievements:
  - Take time to acknowledge and celebrate your successes, no matter how small. Recognize your progress, accomplishments, and milestones along the way.

2. Reward Yourself:
  - Reward yourself for reaching milestones or achieving goals with non-food rewards such as a relaxing bath, a new book, a movie night, or a fun activity you enjoy. Treat yourself to something special as a way of celebrating your hard work and dedication.

3. Practice Gratitude:
  - Cultivate a sense of gratitude for the progress you've made and the positive changes in your life.

Take time to reflect on what you're grateful for and appreciate the effort you've put into achieving your goals.

4. Share Your Successes:

   - Share your successes with others who support and encourage you. Celebrate your achievements with friends, family members, or peers who can share in your joy and provide positive reinforcement.

5. Visualize Your Success:

   - Imagine yourself attaining your objectives and leading the life you have always wanted. Create vision boards, affirmations, or visualization exercises to keep your goals at the forefront of your mind and stay motivated to pursue them.

6. Focus on Progress, Not Perfection:

   - Accept the journey and put more emphasis on advancement than perfection. Celebrate small victories and incremental improvements along the way, and recognize that setbacks and challenges are a normal part of the process.

7. Stay Inspired:

   - Surround yourself with sources of inspiration that will motivate and raise you. Seek out stories, quotes, books, podcasts, or videos that resonate with your goals and aspirations, and draw inspiration from them when you need a boost.

8. Set New Goals:

- Continuously challenge yourself by setting new goals and objectives to strive towards. Setting goals gives you something to work towards and keeps you motivated to continue making progress.

9. Find Joy in the Journey:

- Instead of concentrating only on the outcome, find happiness and contentment in the process of achieving your goals. Embrace the ups and downs, the challenges and triumphs, and the growth and learning that come with striving towards your aspirations.

10. Stay Connected to Your Why:

- Stay connected to your underlying motivations and reasons for pursuing your goals. Remind yourself of why your goals are important to you and how achieving them will enhance your life and well-being.

11. Practice Self-Compassion:

- Treat yourself with kindness and self-compassion, particularly when things are hard. Acknowledge your efforts and progress, and be gentle with yourself when things don't go as planned.

12. Stay Consistent:

- Stay consistent in your efforts and commitments to your goals, even when motivation wanes or obstacles arise. Consistency is key to long-term success and progress towards your aspirations.

By incorporating these strategies into your routine, you can celebrate your successes, stay motivated, and continue making progress towards your goals with enthusiasm and determination. Remember to celebrate every step of the journey and to be proud of how far you've come.

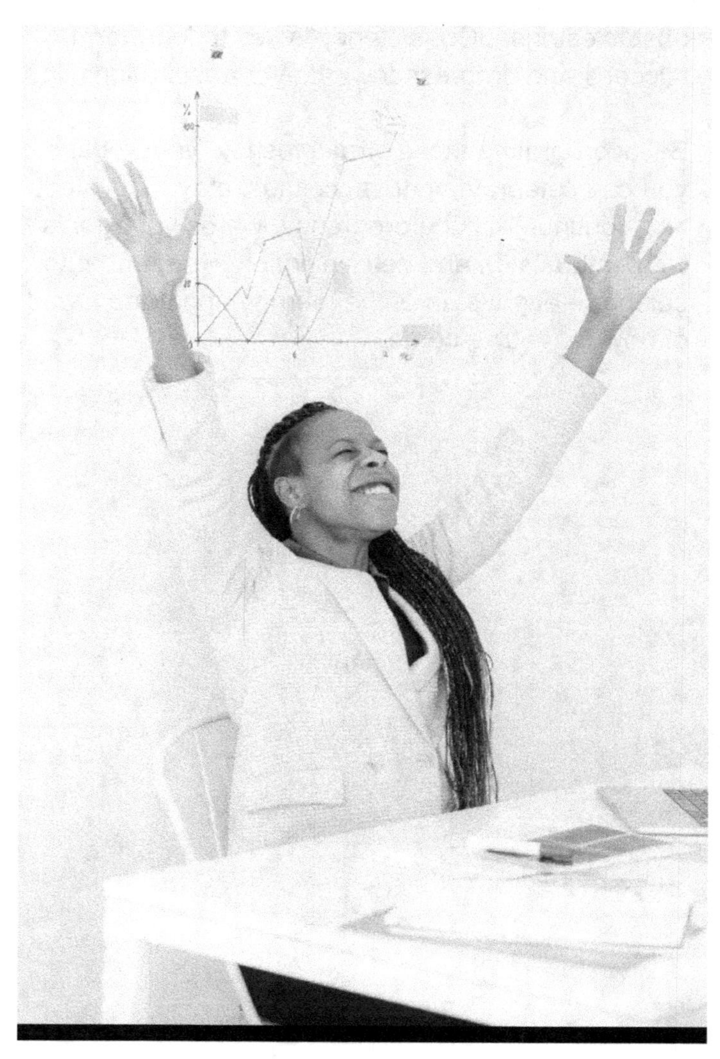

CONCLUSION

In conclusion, prioritizing gut health is essential for overall well-being, particularly for women who often face unique health challenges. This comprehensive guide has provided valuable insights into understanding the importance of gut health, factors affecting it, and practical strategies for maintaining a healthy gut through diet, lifestyle, and mindset adjustments.

We've explored the significance of a balanced diet rich in fiber, probiotics, and prebiotics, along with sample meal plans and recipes tailored to promote gut health. Additionally, we've discussed the influence of lifestyle factors such as stress management, sleep quality, exercise, and how they impact gut health.

Furthermore, we've delved into the intersection between gut health and women's specific health concerns, including hormonal balance, pregnancy, menopause, and how these life stages can affect gastrointestinal function.

By implementing the strategies outlined in this guide, women can empower themselves to take proactive steps towards optimizing their gut health and overall wellness. It's crucial to approach these changes with patience, consistency, and self-compassion, celebrating successes along the way and staying motivated through the journey.

Ultimately, investing in gut health is an investment in long-term vitality, resilience, and vitality. With the knowledge and tools provided in this guide, women can embark on a path towards a healthier, happier, and more vibrant life. Remember, small changes can lead to significant improvements, and every positive choice matters. Here's to a thriving gut and a flourishing life!

FINAL THOUGHTS ON ACHIEVING AND MAINTAINING A HEALTHY GUT FOR WOMEN

In summary, achieving and maintaining a healthy gut is a multifaceted journey that requires a holistic approach encompassing dietary, lifestyle, and mindset adjustments. For women, prioritizing gut health is particularly crucial due to its profound impact on overall well-being and unique health considerations.

To achieve and maintain a healthy gut, women can focus on the following key principles:

1. **Nutrient-Rich Diet:** Embrace a balanced diet rich in fiber, probiotics, and prebiotics to nourish the gut microbiota and support digestive function. A range of entire foods should be included, such as

fruits, vegetables, whole grains, lean meats, and healthy fats.

2. **Lifestyle Optimization:** Manage stress levels through relaxation techniques, prioritize quality sleep, engage in regular physical activity, and avoid unhealthy habits such as smoking and excessive alcohol consumption. These lifestyle factors play a significant role in gut health and overall wellness.

3. **Mindful Eating:** Practice mindful eating by paying attention to hunger and fullness cues, savoring each bite, and avoiding distractions during meals. Cultivate a healthy relationship with food, free from guilt or restriction.

4. **Hormonal Balance:** Recognize the interplay between gut health and hormonal balance, particularly during key life stages such as puberty, menstruation, pregnancy, and menopause. Support hormonal equilibrium through nutrition, stress management, and personalized healthcare.

5. **Consistency and Adaptability:** Strive for consistency in implementing healthy habits while remaining adaptable to life's changes and challenges. Celebrate successes, learn from setbacks, and adjust goals as needed to maintain long-term progress.

By embracing these principles and taking proactive steps to prioritize gut health, women can empower themselves to enhance their overall well-being, vitality, and resilience. Remember, achieving and maintaining a healthy gut is not a destination but a continuous journey of self-care and self-discovery. With dedication, patience, and self-compassion, women can thrive and live their best lives with a healthy gut as their foundation.